Anatomy and Physiology for Nursing and Healthcare Students
at a Glance

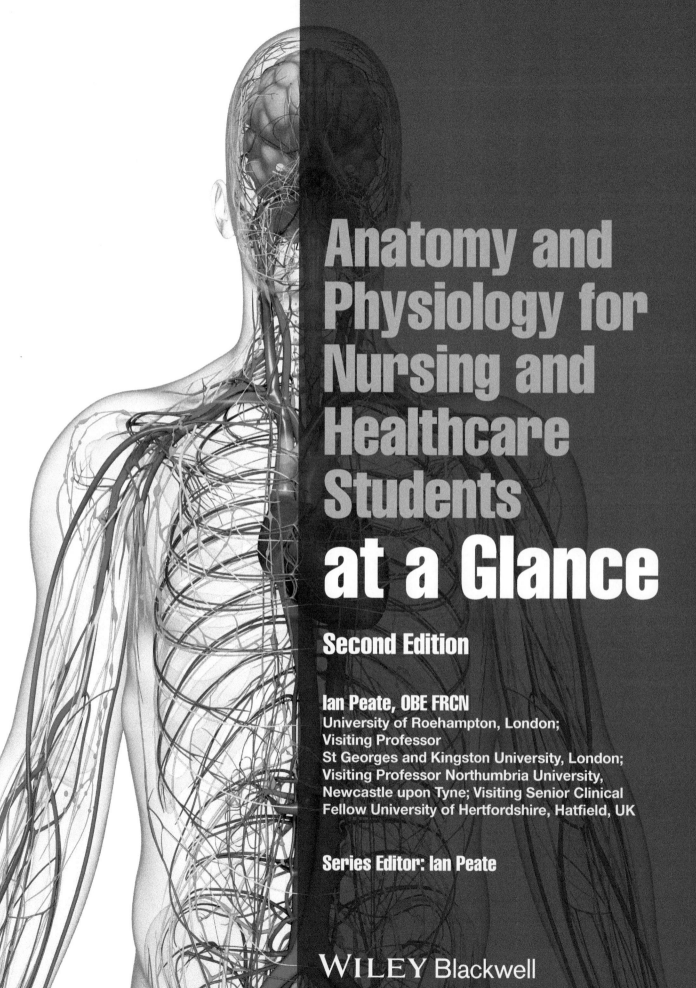

Anatomy and Physiology for Nursing and Healthcare Students

at a Glance

Second Edition

Ian Peate, OBE FRCN
University of Roehampton, London;
Visiting Professor
St Georges and Kingston University, London;
Visiting Professor Northumbria University,
Newcastle upon Tyne; Visiting Senior Clinical
Fellow University of Hertfordshire, Hatfield, UK

Series Editor: Ian Peate

WILEY Blackwell

This edition first published 2022
© 2022 John Wiley & Sons Ltd

Edition History
John Wiley & Sons Ltd (1e, 2015)

Registered Offices
John Wiley & Sons, Inc., 111 River Street, Hoboken, NJ 07030, USA
John Wiley & Sons Ltd, The Atrium, Southern Gate, Chichester, West Sussex, PO19 8SQ, UK

Editorial Office
9600 Garsington Road, Oxford, OX4 2DQ, UK

For details of our global editorial offices, customer services, and more information about Wiley products visit us at www.wiley.com.

Wiley also publishes its books in a variety of electronic formats and by print-on-demand. Some content that appears in standard print versions of this book may not be available in other formats.

Library of Congress Cataloging-in-Publication Data applied for:

ISBN 9781119757207 (paperback)

Cover Design: Wiley
Cover Images: © SEBASTIAN KAULITZKI/Getty Images, PIXOLOGICSTUDIO/ Getty Images

Set in 9.5/11.5pt Minion by Striave, Pondicherry, India
Printed and bound by CPI Group (UK) Ltd, Croydon, CR0 4YY

C9781119757207_261023

Contents

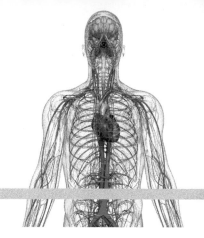

Preface

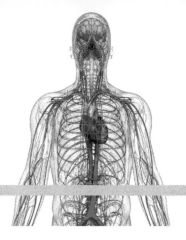

I am delighted to have been asked to provide a second edition of *Anatomy and Physiology for Nursing and Healthcare Students at a Glance*. This popular revision aid has retained the user-friendly approach that includes bite-sized pieces of information and full-colour diagrams that help students retain, recall and apply facts to their practice.

All health and care providers aim to offer care that is safe and effective. In order to care effectively for people (sick or well), it is essential to have an understanding of and insight into anatomy and physiology.

The human body is composed of organic and inorganic molecules organised at a variety of structural levels; despite this, an individual should be seen and treated in a holistic manner. If the healthcare professional is to provide appropriate and timely care, it is essential that they are able to recognise illness, take prompt action to deliver effective treatment and refer appropriately, ensuring that the person they offer care and support to is at the centre of all that they do.

Healthcare professionals are required to demonstrate a sound knowledge of anatomy and physiology with the intention of providing safe and effective nursing care. This is often assessed as a part of a programme of study using a number of assessment techniques. The overall aim of this concise text is to provide an overview of anatomy and physiology and the related biological sciences that can help to develop your practical skills and improve your knowledge with the aim of you becoming a caring, knowledgeable and compassionate provider of care. It is anticipated that you will be able to deliver increasingly complex care for the people you care for when you understand how the body functions.

As you begin to appreciate how people respond or adapt to pathophysiological changes and stressors, you will be able to understand that people (regardless of their age) all have unique biological needs. The integration and application of evidence-based theory to practice is a key component of effective and safe healthcare. However, this goal cannot be achieved without an understanding of anatomy and physiology.

An additional chapter has been introduced, Anatomical Terms, emphasising the importance of understanding and using the correct anatomical terminology when making a description of body parts as a shared method of communicating between health and care staff. This new edition also includes clinical practice points which aim to encourage readers to relate the theoretical concepts described to practice.

Anatomy is associated with the function of a living organism and as such it is almost always inseparable from physiology. Physiology is the science dealing with the study of the function of cells, tissues, organs and organisms; it is the study of life.

Ian Peate
London

Abbreviations

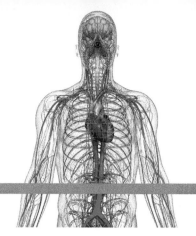

ACTH	Adrenocorticotrophic hormone	**HR**	Heart rate
ADH	Antidiuretic hormone	**K⁺**	Potassium
ANP	Atrial natriuretic peptide	**kPa**	Kilopascal
ANS	Autonomic nervous system	**Mg²⁺**	Magnesium
ATP	Adenosine triphosphate	**mmHg**	Millimetres of mercury
AV	Atrioventricular	**mRNA**	Messenger ribonucleic acid
BBB	Blood–brain barrier	**Na⁺**	Sodium
BP	Blood pressure	**NH₃**	Ammonia
Ca²⁺	Calcium	**O₂**	Oxygen
CCK	Cholecystokinin	**PCA**	Posterior cerebral artery
Cl	Chloride	**PCO₂**	Partial pressure of carbon dioxide
CNS	Central nervous system	**PCT**	Proximal convoluted tubule
CRH	Corticotrophin-releasing hormone	**pH**	A measure of the acidity or basicity of an aqueous solution
CSF	Cerebrospinal fluid		
CO₂	Carbon dioxide	**PNS**	Parasympathetic nervous system
CRC	Cardioregulatory centre	**PO₂**	Partial pressure of oxygen
CSF	Cerebrospinal fluid	**PRH**	Prolactin-releasing hormone
DNA	Deoxyribonucleic acid	**RBC**	Red blood cell
EPO	Erythropoietin	**RER**	Rough endoplasmic reticulum
FSH	Follicle-stimulating hormone	**RNA**	Ribonucleic acid
GH	Growth hormone	**rRNA**	Ribosomal ribonucleic acid
GHRIF	Growth hormone release-inhibiting factor	**SA**	Sinoatrial
H⁺	Hydrogen	**SER**	Smooth endoplasmic reticulum
H₂O	Water	**SNS**	Sympathetic nervous system
Hb	Haemoglobin	**tRNA**	Transfer ribonucleic acid
HCG	Human chorionic gonadotrophin	**TSH**	Thyroid-stimulating hormone
HCL	Hydrochloric acid	**WBC**	White blood cell

Acknowledgements

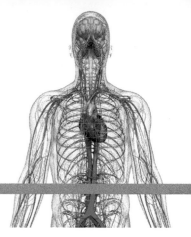

Ian would like to thank his partner Jussi Lahtinen and also Mrs Frances Cohen for all their support and encouragement.

How to use your revision guide and the companion website

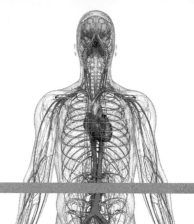

Features contained within your revision guide

Each topic is presented in a double-page spread with clear, easy-to-follow diagrams supported by succinct explanatory text.

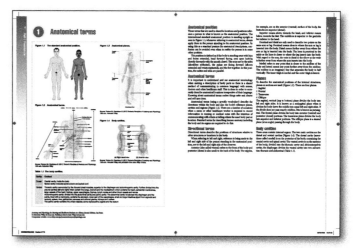

Don't forget to visit the companion website for this book:

www.wiley.com/go/peate/anatomyandphysiology

This hosts interactive multiple-choice questions for every chapter designed to enhance your learning.

Foundations

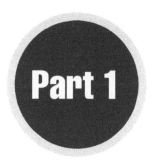

Part 1

Chapters

1 Anatomical terms

Figure 1.1   The standard anatomical position.

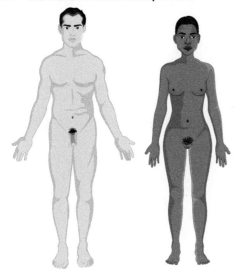

Figure 1.2   Anatomical terms.

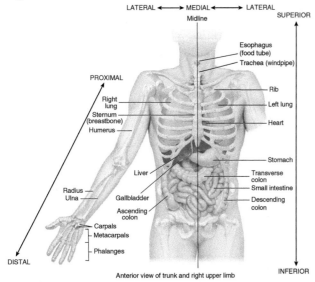

LATERAL ←→ MEDIAL ←→ LATERAL
Midline
SUPERIOR

PROXIMAL

Esophagus (food tube)
Trachea (windpipe)
Rib
Left lung
Heart

Right lung
Sternum (breastbone)
Humerus

Stomach
Transverse colon
Small intestine
Descending colon

Liver
Radius
Ulna
Gallbladder
Ascending colon

Carpals
Metacarpals
Phalanges

DISTAL
Anterior view of trunk and right upper limb
INFERIOR

Source: Tortora GJ, Derrickson B. (2017) Tortora's Principles of Anatomy and Physiology, 15th edn. Hoboken: Wiley

Figure 1.3   Anatomical planes.

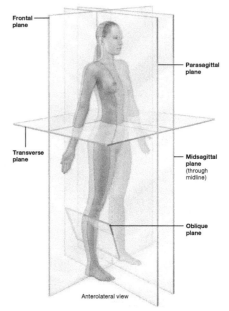

Frontal plane
Parasagittal plane
Transverse plane
Midsagittal plane (through midline)
Oblique plane
Anterolateral view

Source: Tortora GJ, Derrickson B. (2017) Tortora's Principles of Anatomy and Physiology, 15th edn. Hoboken: Wiley

Figure 1.4   Body cavities.

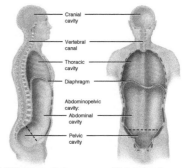

Cranial cavity
Vertebral canal
Thoracic cavity
Diaphragm
Abdominopelvic cavity:
Abdominal cavity
Pelvic cavity

(a) Right lateral view   (b) Anterior view

Source: Tortora GJ, Derrickson B. (2017) Tortora's Principles of Anatomy and Physiology, 15th edn. Hoboken: Wiley, with permission from John Wiley & Sons.

Table 1.1 The body cavities.

Cavity	Content
Dorsal	Cranial cavity: holds the brain Spinal cavity: includes spinal column and spinal cord
Ventral	Thoracic cavity: surrounded by the ribs and chest muscles, superior to the diaphragm and abdominopelvic cavity. Further divided into the pleural cavities (left and right) which contain the lungs, bronchi and the mediastinum which contains the heart, pericardial membranes, large vessels of the heart, trachea, upper oesophagus, thymus, lymph nodes and other blood vessels and nerves Abdominopelvic cavity: divided into the abdominal cavity and pelvic cavity. The abdominal cavity: is between the diaphragm and the pelvis, lined with a membrane, contains the stomach, lower part of the oesophagus, small and large intestines (apart from sigmoid and rectum), spleen, liver, gallbladder, pancreas and adrenal glands, kidneys and ureters. The pelvic cavity: contains the urinary bladder, some reproductive organs and the rectum

Anatomy and Physiology for Nursing and Healthcare Students at a Glance, Second Edition. Ian Peate.
© 2022 John Wiley & Sons Ltd. Published 2022 by John Wiley & Sons Ltd.
Companion website: www.wiley.com/go/peate/anatomyandphysiology

Anatomical position

Those terms that are used to describe locations and positions reference a person in what is known as the anatomical position. The international standard anatomical position is standing upright as seen in Figure 1.1; whenever referring to anatomical terms, always apply them to the person standing in the anatomical position. By using this as a standard posture for anatomical descriptions, confusion can be avoided even when in reality the person is in some other position.

The position is defined as if the body is standing erect with hips and knees extended, head forward facing, eyes open looking directly forwards with the mouth closed. The arms are by the sides (shoulders adducted), the palms are facing forward (elbows extended and wrists supinated), and the feet together. In this position, the radius and ulna are parallel.

Anatomical terms

It is important to understand and use anatomical terminology when making a description of body parts so there is a shared method of communicating (a common language) with nurses, doctors and other healthcare staff. This is done in order to accurately describe anatomical locations irrespective of their language. Knowing about anatomical terms makes things safer and clearer and will save time.

Anatomical terms (using a specific vocabulary) describe the directions within the body and also the body's reference planes, cavities and regions (Figure 1.2). There are a number of occasions when a nurse or other healthcare worker is required to record information in nursing or medical notes with the intention of communicating with others or telling others the exact body part or location. Standard terms for describing human anatomy including the body and its organs are required to do this.

Directional terms

Directional terms describe the positions of structures relative to other structures or locations in the body.

When referring to left and right, reference is being made to the left and right side of the person standing in the anatomical position, not to the left and right side of the observer.

Anterior (also called ventral) refers to the front of the body and posterior (dorsal is also used) to the back of the body. The nipples, for example, are on the anterior (ventral) surface of the body, the buttocks are superior (dorsal).

Superior means above, towards the head, and inferior means below, towards the feet. The umbilicus is superior to the genitalia but inferior to the head.

Proximal and distal are only used to describe two points on the same arm or leg. Proximal means close to where the arm or leg is inserted into the body. Distal means further away from where the arm or leg is inserted into the body. The knee is proximal to the ankle as the knee is closer to where the leg inserts into the body. With regard to the arm, the wrist is distal to the elbow as the wrist is further away from where the arm inserts into the body.

Medial refers to any point that is closer to the midline of the body and lateral means any point further away from the midline. The midline is an imaginary line that separates the body in half vertically. The inner thigh is medial and the outer thigh is lateral.

Planes

To describe the anatomical positions of the internal structures, planes or sections are used (Figure 1.3). There are four planes.
1 Sagittal
2 Frontal
3 Transverse
4 Oblique

The sagittal, vertical (top to bottom) plane divides the body into left and right sides. It is known as a midsagittal plane when it divides the body down the middle into equal left and right sides. If the divide does not pass exactly midline, this is known as parasagittal. The frontal plane divides the body into anterior (ventral) and posterior (dorsal) portions. The transverse plane divides the body into superior and inferior portions. The oblique plane is a slanted plane (at an angle) passing through the body.

Body cavities

These areas contain internal organs. The two main cavities are the dorsal and ventral cavities (Figure 1.4). The dorsal cavity (sometimes called caudal) is on the posterior of the body, containing the cranial cavity and spinal cavity. The ventral cavity is on the anterior of the body, divided into the thoracic cavity and abdominopelvic cavity; the diaphragm divides the ventral cavity into two subcavities: thoracic and abdominal (Table 1.1).

2 Genetics and genomics

Figure 2.1 DNA and RNA.

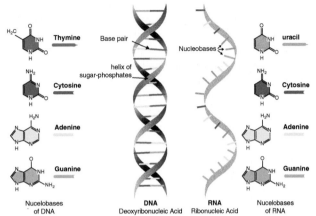

Thymine

Base pair

Nucleobases

uracil

Cytosine

Cytosine

helix of sugar-phosphates

Adenine

Adenine

Guanine

Guanine

Nucelobases of DNA

DNA Deoxyribonucleic Acid

RNA Ribonucleic Acid

Nucelobases of RNA

Table 2.1 Types of RNA.

Type of RNA	Description
Messenger RNA (mRNA)	Copies portions of genetic code, a process known as transcription, and transports these copies to ribosomes, the cellular factories that facilitate the production of proteins from this code
Transfer RNA (tRNA)	Responsible for bringing amino acids, basic protein building blocks, to these protein factories, in response to the coded instructions introduced by the mRNA. This protein-building process is called translation
Ribosomal RNA (rRNA)	The protein builder of the cell, without which protein production would not occur

Figure 2.2 Mitosis.

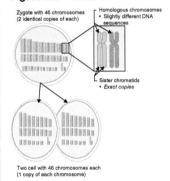

Zygote with 46 chromosomes (2 identical copies of each)

Homologous chromosomes
• Slightly different DNA sequences

Sister chromatids
• Exact copies

Two cell with 46 chromosomes each (1 copy of each chromosome)

Figure 2.3 Meiosis.

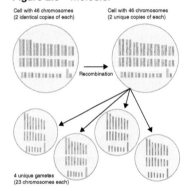

Cell with 46 chromosomes (2 identical copies of each)

Cell with 46 chromosomes (2 unique copies of each)

Recombination

4 unique gametes (23 chromosomes each)

Figure 2.4 Fertilisation.

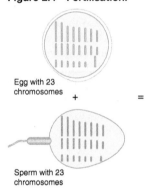

Egg with 23 chromosomes

+

Sperm with 23 chromosomes

=

Zygote with 46 chromosomes

Anatomy and Physiology for Nursing and Healthcare Students at a Glance, Second Edition. Ian Peate.
© 2022 John Wiley & Sons Ltd. Published 2022 by John Wiley & Sons Ltd.
Companion website: www.wiley.com/go/peate/anatomyandphysiology

Genetics is the study of the way particular features or diseases are inherited through genes passed down from one generation to the next. The idea of having a single gene for this or a single gene for that (determining fate) is not a good way of describing the complexity of genes. There are groups of genes that work together, influenced by a variety of environmental and other factors. The genome can be seen as the body's instruction manual, with a copy of it in almost every healthy cell in the body. The study of the genome and the technologies that are required to analyse and interpret it is known as genomics.

DNA and RNA

Both deoxyribonucleic acid (DNA) and ribonucleic acid (RNA) are made of nucleotides (bases) which are the building blocks, responsible for the storage and reading of genetic information that underpins all life. DNA encodes all genetic information, also acting as a biological store allowing the blueprint of life to be passed between generations. RNA reads and then decodes what is stored. This is a multistep process with specialised RNAs for each step (Table 2.1).

DNA and RNA are nucleic acids, known as linear polymers, consisting of sugars, phosphates and bases, but there are differences between the two. The differences permit the two molecules to work together, fulfilling essential roles. See Figure 2.1 for the differences. The complementary base pairs in DNA are adenine ('A'), thymine ('T'), guanine ('G') and cytosine ('C') and RNA shares adenine ('A'), guanine ('G') and cytosine ('C') with DNA, but contains uracil ('U') instead of thymine (Figure 2.1).

Molecules in DNA have an even and uniform shape while in RNA they are uneven and diverse shapes. DNA molecules are made up of millions of nucleotides and RNA molecules are usually smaller, composed of hundreds to a few thousand nucleotides.

Mitosis, meiosis and fertilisation

The human cell usually has 46 chromosomes: 44 autosomes, which are paired, and two sex chromosomes, usually specifying whether someone is male (usually XY) or female (usually XX). Autosomes, known as homologous chromosomes, have all of the same genes arranged in the same order, However, there are small differences in the DNA letters of the genes.

Mitosis occurs when cells divide to make more cells or reproductive cells (meiosis), and when reproductive cells join to make a new individual (fertilisation).

Mitosis

Prior to a cell dividing to make two cells, all of its chromosomes are copied, known as sister chromatids. Until cell division, the copies stay connected with each other by their middles (centromeres.) Upon cell division, the copies are pulled apart, each new cell getting one identical copy of each chromosome. Every cell has an identical set of chromosomes (see Figure 2.2).

Meiosis

When egg and sperm cells form, they go through a type of cell division called meiosis. Meiosis reduces the number of chromosomes by half as well as creating genetic diversity. The cell copies each chromosome, unlike in mitosis, homologous chromosome pairs align, exchanging pieces (recombination). Recombination increases genetic diversity by adding pieces of slightly different chromosomes together. The recombined homologous chromosomes are divided into two daughter cells. Then the sister chromatids are pulled apart into a total of four reproductive cells. Each of these cells has one copy each of 23 chromosomes; all possess a unique combination of gene variations (Figure 2.3).

Fertilisation

Egg and sperm cells have 23 chromosomes each, half as many chromosomes as regular cells. Through the process of fertilisation, egg and sperm join, making a cell with 46 chromosomes (23 pairs), a zygote. For each chromosomal pair, one homologous chromosome came from each parent. Genes are arranged in the same order but there are small variations in the DNA letters of those genes (Figure 2.4).

Clinical practice point

Nurses and other healthcare professionals are ideally placed to offer and promote genetic and genomic healthcare as they highlight health promotion, prevention, screening, patient, family and community relationships.

A genetic disorder is a disease caused by a change in the DNA sequence away from the normal sequence. Genetic disorders can be caused by a mutation in one gene, by mutations in multiple genes, by a combination of gene mutations and environmental factors, or damage to chromosomes.

3 Homeostasis

Figure 3.1 Components of a negative feedback system.

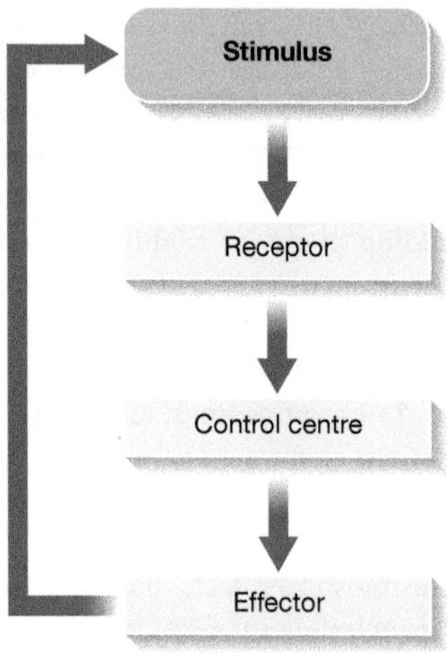

Stimulus

↓

Receptor

↓

Control centre

↓

Effector

Figure 3.2 Negative feedback – raised blood pressure.

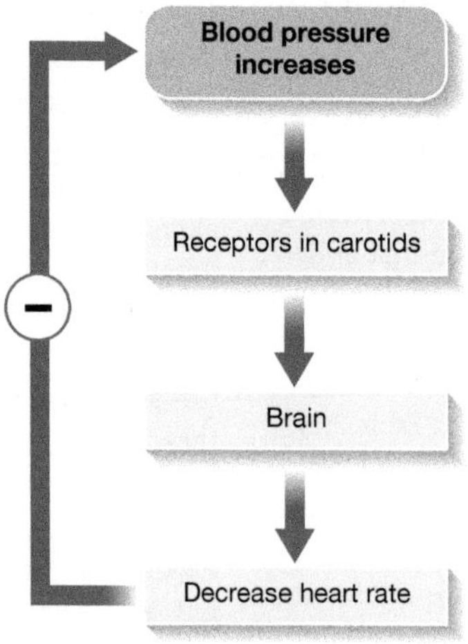

Blood pressure increases

↓

Receptors in carotids

↓

Brain

↓

Decrease heart rate

(−)

Figure 3.3 Negative feedback – raised temperature.

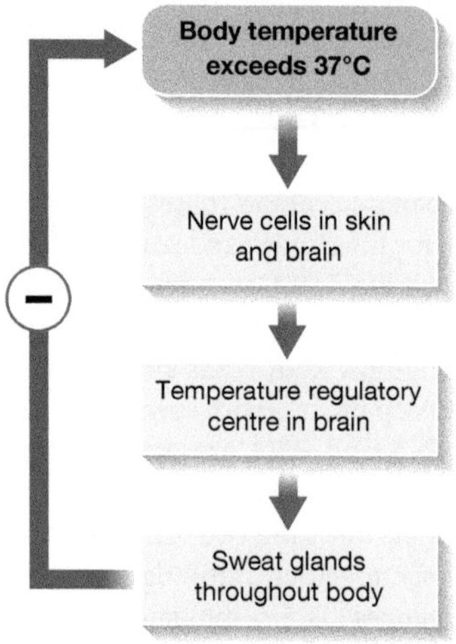

Body temperature exceeds 37°C

↓

Nerve cells in skin and brain

↓

Temperature regulatory centre in brain

↓

Sweat glands throughout body

(−)

Figure 3.4 Positive feedback of childbirth.

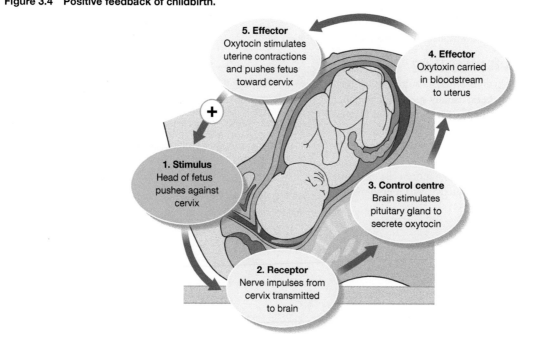

5. Effector
Oxytocin stimulates uterine contractions and pushes fetus toward cervix

4. Effector
Oxytoxin carried in bloodstream to uterus

1. Stimulus
Head of fetus pushes against cervix

3. Control centre
Brain stimulates pituitary gland to secrete oxytocin

2. Receptor
Nerve impulses from cervix transmitted to brain

(+)

Anatomy and Physiology for Nursing and Healthcare Students at a Glance, Second Edition. Ian Peate.
© 2022 John Wiley & Sons Ltd. Published 2022 by John Wiley & Sons Ltd.
Companion website: www.wiley.com/go/peate/anatomyandphysiology

Homeostasis

Homeostasis is an important physiological concept and can be defined as the ability of the body or a cell to seek and maintain a condition of equilibrium within its internal environment when dealing with external changes. It is a state of equilibrium for the body. Homeostasis allows the organs of the body to function effectively in a broad range of conditions.

All the organs and organ systems of the human body work together in harmony and are closely regulated by the nervous and endocrine systems. The nervous system controls almost all body activities and the endocrine system secretes hormones that regulate these activities. Working together, the organ systems supply body cells with all the substances needed and also eliminate waste. They also keep temperature, pH, blood glucose and other conditions at just the right levels required to support life processes.

- Temperature at 36.5 °C
- Blood glucose – 4–8 mmol/L
- pH of the blood – 7.4

Feedback mechanisms

There are a variety of feedback mechanisms used by the body to regulate internal systems. There are three fundamental elements associated with the feedback system: a receptor, a control centre and an effector (Figure 3.1). The effector may be a muscle, organs or another structure that receives messages indicating a reaction is required.

Receptor

The receptor senses changes in the internal environment, relaying information to the control centre. Specific nerve endings in the skin, for example, sense a change in temperature, detecting changes such as a sudden increase or fall in body temperature.

Control centre

The brain is the control centre, receiving information from the receptor and interpreting the information, and then sending information to the effector. The output could be nerve impulses or hormones or other chemical signals.

Effector

An effector is a body system, for example, the skin, blood vessels or the blood, that receives the information from the control centre, producing a response to the condition. For example, in the regulation of body temperature by our skin (if it drops below normal), the hypothalamus acts as the control centre, which receives input from the skin. The output from the control centre goes to the skeletal muscles via nerves to initiate shivering and this raises body temperature.

Negative feedback

Most body systems work on negative feedback. Negative feedback ensures that, in any control system, changes are reversed and then returned back to the set level. An example might be, if the blood pressure increases, then receptors in the carotid arteries detect this change in blood pressure and relay a message to the brain. The brain will cause the heart to beat more slowly and, by doing this, work towards decreasing the blood pressure. Decreasing heart rate has a negative effect on blood pressure (Figure 3.2). Another example of negative feedback is regulation of body temperature at a constant 37 °C. If we get too hot, blood vessels in the skin vasodilate and heat is lost and we cool down. If we get too cold, blood vessels in the skin vasoconstrict, we lose less heat and the body warms up. The negative feedback system therefore ensures that homeostasis is maintained (Figure 3.3).

Positive feedback

This is the mechanism used by the body to enhance an output needed to maintain homeostasis. Positive feedback mechanisms push levels out of normal ranges. While this process can be beneficial, it is rarely used by the body because of the risk of the increased stimuli becoming out of control.

An example of positive feedback is the release of oxytocin (a hormone) to increase and keep the contractions of childbirth happening as long as needed for the child's birth. Contractions of the uterus are stimulated by oxytocin, produced in the pituitary gland in the brain, and the secretion of it is increased by positive feedback, increasing the strength of the contractions (Figure 3.4).

Another example of positive feedback occurs in lactation, during which the mother produces milk for her child. During pregnancy, levels of prolactin (a hormone) increase. Prolactin normally stimulates milk production but during pregnancy, progesterone inhibits milk production. At birth, when the placenta is released from the uterus, levels of progesterone drop and as a result, milk production flows. As the infant feeds, its suckling stimulates the breast, promoting further release of prolactin, producing even more. This positive feedback ensures the infant has sufficient milk during feeding. When the baby is weaned and is no longer breast feeding, stimulation stops, with prolactin in the mother's blood returning to pre-breastfeeding levels.

Clinical practice point

Respiratory system: a high concentration of carbon dioxide in the blood triggers faster breathing. The lungs exhale more frequently, which removes carbon dioxide from the body faster.

Excretory system: a low level of water in the blood triggers retention of water by the kidneys. The kidneys produce more concentrated urine, therefore less water is lost from the body.

Endocrine system: a high concentration of glucose in the blood triggers secretion of insulin by the pancreas. Insulin, a hormone, helps cells absorb glucose from the blood.

4 Fluid compartments

Figure 4.1   Body water content.

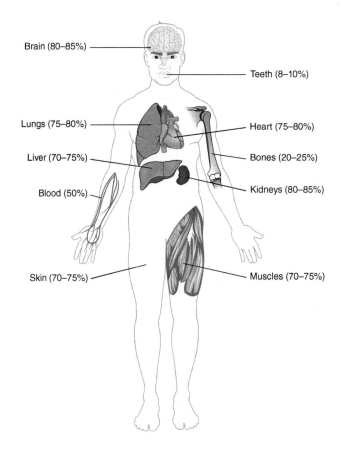

Brain (80–85%)

Teeth (8–10%)

Lungs (75–80%)

Heart (75–80%)

Liver (70–75%)

Bones (20–25%)

Blood (50%)

Kidneys (80–85%)

Skin (70–75%)

Muscles (70–75%)

Figure 4.2   Fluid compartments.

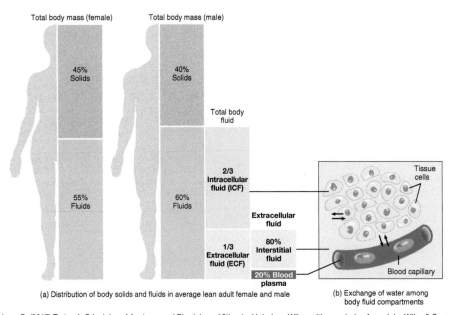

Total body mass (female)

Total body mass (male)

45%
Solids

40%
Solids

Total body
fluid

2/3
Intracellular
fluid (ICF)

Tissue
cells

55%
Fluids

60%
Fluids

Extracellular
fluid

1/3
Extracellular
fluid (ECF)

80%
Interstitial
fluid

20% Blood
plasma

Blood capillary

(a) Distribution of body solids and fluids in average lean adult female and male

(b) Exchange of water among
body fluid compartments

Source: Tortora GJ, Derrickson B. (2017) Tortora's Principles of Anatomy and Physiology, 15th edn. Hoboken: Wiley, with permission from John Wiley & Sons.

Anatomy and Physiology for Nursing and Healthcare Students at a Glance, Second Edition. Ian Peate.
© 2022 John Wiley & Sons Ltd. Published 2022 by John Wiley & Sons Ltd.
Companion website: www.wiley.com/go/peate/anatomyandphysiology

The ability to maintain an adequate fluid balance is essential to health. Inadequate fluid intake or excessive fluid loss can lead to dehydration, which may impact negatively on renal and cardiac performance and electrolyte function. Regulating the volume and composition of body fluids, controlling how they are distributed throughout the body and balancing body fluid are critical when maintaining homeostasis and health.

Body water

A body fluid is a substance, usually a liquid, produced by the body that comprises water and dissolved solutes. Body fluids are dilute water solutions. Humans are predominantly made up of water, which ranges from around 75% of body mass in infants to approximately 50–60% in adult men and women and in old age as low as 45%. Body water varies with the amount of adipose tissue that the body stores. As the amount of adipose tissue increases, percentage of body water falls. Women tend to store more adipose tissue than men.

The brain and kidneys have the highest proportions of water, composed of 80–85% of their masses. The teeth, in contrast, have the lowest proportion of water at 8–10% (Figure 4.1).

Location of body fluids

Body fluids are present in two main 'compartments': inside cells and outside cells (Figure 4.2). Around two-thirds of body fluid is intracellular fluid (ICF) or cytosol, the fluid which is located within cells. The other one-third is extracellular fluid (ECF), outside cells, and includes all other body fluids. Approximately 80% of the ECF is interstitial fluid, which fills the microscopic spaces between tissue cells; 20% of the ECF is blood plasma (the liquid component of blood). Other extracellular fluids include interstitial fluid, which includes the lymph in lymphatic vessels; cerebrospinal fluid in the nervous system; synovial fluid in joints; aqueous humor and vitreous body in the eyes; endolymph and perilymph in the ears and pleural, pericardial and peritoneal fluids located between serous membranes.

Intracellular fluid

Around two-thirds of the body's fluid is intracellular in the adult, contained within more than 100 trillion cells; this amounts to approximately 28 litres for an average 70 kg male. These vast numbers of cells are not physically united; the ICF compartment is a virtual compartment. These are small discontinuous collections of fluid but from a physiological perspective, intracellular fluid is considered as if it were one single compartment.

Extracellular fluid

Extracellular fluid is located outside cells, surrounding them. Effective functioning of body cells depends on the precise regulation of the composition of their surrounding fluid. As the ECF surrounds the cells of the body, it serves as the body's internal environment. The space that surrounds the entire body is the external environment.

Extracellular fluid declines as we age and is more readily lost from the body than the ICF. ECF is usually subdivided into a number of smaller compartments that are located in the intravascular and interstitial compartments or spaces. The intravascular compartment comprises the fluid within the blood vessels (the plasma volume). In an average adult blood volume amounts to 5–6 litres, approximately 3 litres of which is plasma. The interstitial fluid is the fluid in the 'gaps' between the cells and outside the blood vessels; this includes lymph fluid, sometimes called the 'third space'. Transcellular fluid is fluid contained within particular cavities of the body and digestive secretions that are separated by a layer of epithelium from the interstitial compartment. Transcellular fluid is akin to interstitial fluid and often this is considered to be a part of interstitial volume. The transcellular fluid amounts to around 1 litre.

Maintaining fluid balance

Fluid balance is the balance between the volume of fluid taken in and the volume of fluid the body excretes. Optimal hydration is achieved when the volume of fluid taken in matches the volume of fluid excreted. Maintaining fluid balance is primarily accomplished through renal activity. Fluid intake and urine output are the key processes for maintaining fluid balance. A fall in circulating plasma volume, for example due to haemorrhage, can affect bodily functions such as oxygen delivery to the tissues and cells.

Body fluid movement

Fluid within the body can be thought of as separated into numerous functional compartments that are divided by semi-permeable membranes permitting free movement of water but not of certain classes of solutes. In a healthy individual, fluid is divided between these functional compartments in specific ratios. The force that allows fluids to move between the body's fluid compartments is a difference between the compartments' relative osmolarity. Fluid moves between compartments until their relative osmolarity is balanced and a new steady state is achieved. Changes in osmolarity usually impact the ECF first as this is the compartment immediately in contact with the external environment. Once the ECF osmolarity changes, water moves into or out of the intracellular compartment within minutes, until a new osmolar equilibrium is established between the ECF and ICF.

Clinical practice point

Fluid balance charts (records) are a critical component of patient care and the duty for keeping fluid balance charts lies with nurses. All nurses are required to perform a thorough hydration assessment so as to plan and deliver individualised patient care. During handover and between shifts, a report on the patient's fluid intake and output (fluid balance information) should be discussed in order to identify and prevent deterioration.

⑤ Cells and organelles

Figure 5.1 Structures located within body cells.

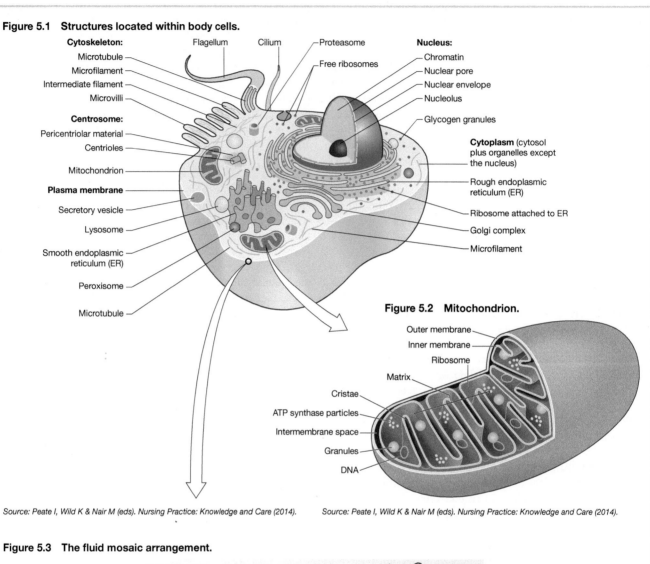

Cytoskeleton:
Microtubule
Microfilament
Intermediate filament
Microvilli

Centrosome:
Pericentriolar material
Centrioles

Mitochondrion

Plasma membrane

Secretory vesicle

Lysosome

Smooth endoplasmic reticulum (ER)

Peroxisome

Microtubule

Flagellum
Cilium
Proteasome
Free ribosomes

Nucleus:
Chromatin
Nuclear pore
Nuclear envelope
Nucleolus

Glycogen granules

Cytoplasm (cytosol plus organelles except the nucleus)

Rough endoplasmic reticulum (ER)

Ribosome attached to ER

Golgi complex

Microfilament

Source: Peate I, Wild K & Nair M (eds). Nursing Practice: Knowledge and Care (2014).

Figure 5.2 Mitochondrion.

Outer membrane
Inner membrane
Ribosome
Matrix
Cristae
ATP synthase particles
Intermembrane space
Granules
DNA

Source: Peate I, Wild K & Nair M (eds). Nursing Practice: Knowledge and Care (2014).

Figure 5.3 The fluid mosaic arrangement.

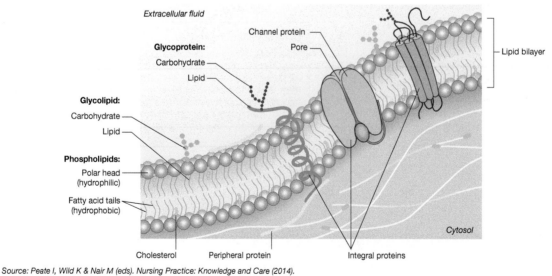

Extracellular fluid

Glycoprotein:
Carbohydrate
Lipid

Glycolipid:
Carbohydrate
Lipid

Phospholipids:
Polar head (hydrophilic)
Fatty acid tails (hydrophobic)

Channel protein
Pore

Lipid bilayer

Cholesterol
Peripheral protein
Integral proteins

Cytosol

Source: Peate I, Wild K & Nair M (eds). Nursing Practice: Knowledge and Care (2014).

Anatomy and Physiology for Nursing and Healthcare Students at a Glance, Second Edition. Ian Peate.
© 2022 John Wiley & Sons Ltd. Published 2022 by John Wiley & Sons Ltd.
Companion website: www.wiley.com/go/peate/anatomyandphysiology

Table 5.1 Common elements in the body.

Element	Role
Oxygen (O_2)	Component of water (H_2O) and most organic molecules, used to produce adenosine triphosphate (ATP), an energy provider within the cell
Carbon dioxide (CO_2)	Vital component of all organic molecules, such as carbohydrates, lipids, proteins and nucleic acids (deoxyribonucleic acid [DNA] and ribonucleic acid [RNA])
Hydrogen (H)	Element of water and most organic molecules
Nitrogen (N)	Principal element of all proteins and nucleic acids
Calcium (Ca)	Required for effective mineralisation of bones and teeth; the ionised form (Ca^{2+}) is needed for blood clotting and muscle contraction
Phosphorus (P)	Component of nucleic acids and ATP. Found in healthy bones and teeth
Potassium (K)	In its ionised form (K^+) is the most abundant cation in intracellular fluid; required for the generation of electrical activity in the nerve axon (action potentials)
Sulfur (S)	Present in a number of proteins and some vitamins
Chloride (Cl)	The ionised form (Cl^-) is the most abundant anion in extracellular fluid: crucial for maintaining water balance
Magnesium (Mg)	Necessary for action of many enzymes
Iron (Fe)	Essential component of haemoglobin (Hb), the oxygen-carrying protein in red blood cells

Cells are the basic living, structural and functional units of the body. It is generally agreed that the cell is the smallest independent, living structure, varying in size from 7.5 micrometres (for example, a red blood cell) to 150 micrometres (such as an ovum). Cells undertake a number of functions that help each system participate in homeostasis (see Chapter 3). All cells share key structures and functions that provide support for their intense activity.

Humans are multicellular beings. Each cell can take in nutrients, convert those nutrients into energy, undertake specialised functions and reproduce as required. Cells arise from existing cells, as one cell divides into two identical cells. The different types of cells carry out unique roles that support homeostasis and provide assistance for the many functional capabilities of the human organism.

Cell structure and function are closely related. Cells carry out an assortment of chemical reactions, creating and maintaining life processes. The types of chemical reactions within specialised cellular structures are co-ordinated to maintain life in a cell, tissue, organ, system and organism.

While a cell is the smallest living structure within the body, each cell is made up of smaller components, called atoms. Atoms of the same type form elements. See Table 5.1 for the most common elements found in the body

Components of a cell

There are more than 100 trillion cells in the average adult human body. Cells are the basic, living, structural and functional units of the body. The study of cells is known as cytology. Figure 5.1 offers an overview of the structures usually found in body cells. The cell can be divided into three main parts: cell membrane (plasma membrane), cytoplasm and nucleus.

Cell membrane

The cell (or plasma) membrane forms the external boundary of the cell; it is flexible yet strong and contains the cytoplasm of the cell. This gives it its shape; the membrane protects the cell's contents, keeping the contents within the cell. The cell's internal environment can thereby be held stable and distinct from the external environment. The cell membrane is selectively permeable, regulating the movement of molecules into and out of the cell.

The membrane is made up of two layers of fat molecules, containing phosphate, called phospholipids, which form a fluid framework for the cell membrane. Embedded in the phospholipid bilayer are protein and sugar molecules distributed in a mosaic pattern, described as the fluid mosaic model (Figure 5.3).

Cytoplasm

This is made up of all the cellular content between the plasma membrane and the nucleus, with two components: the cytosol and organelles, the tiny structures that perform distinct functions in the cell. Organelles are specialised structures located within the cell; they have characteristic shapes and perform specific functions in cellular growth, maintenance and reproduction. The numbers and types of organelles vary between cell types and although they have different functions, organelles can help to maintain cellular homeostasis. Key organelles include the endoplasmic reticulum, ribosomes, mitochondria, Golgi apparatus, lysosomes, peroxisomes, centrosomes, cilia and flagella (see Figures 5.1 and 5.2). Cytoplasm is enclosed within the cell membrane; it is the substance that fills the cell and is the living material of the cell composed primarily of cytosol, as well as sugars, proteins, ions, molecules and enzymes that are used in cellular activity. All the cell's organelles are suspended in the cytosol and are held together by a fatty membrane.

Nucleus

It is the nucleus that contains genes (these are located on chromosomes) which control every organelle in the cytoplasm; genes within the nucleus also control cell reproduction. The function of the nucleus is to maintain the integrity of the genes and control the activities of the cell; it does this by regulating gene expression. The nucleus is therefore the control centre of the cell. The nucleus is surrounded by a membrane, enclosing a particular type of cytoplasm called nucleoplasm. The majority of cells contain a single nucleus but there are some cells that have none, for example, mature red blood cells. Skeletal muscle cells have multiple nuclei.

The nuclear pores control the transportation of substances between the nucleus and the cytoplasm. Smaller molecules and ions move through the pores passively by diffusion. The majority of larger molecules, for example RNAs and proteins, are unable to use the passive mechanism and have to be actively transported. The molecules are recognised and selectively transported through the nuclear pore into or out of the nucleus. Nucleoli are responsible for the synthesis of large amounts of protein, for example muscle and liver cells.

Clinical practice point

Body cells have a number of important features, reproducing when and where needed, in the right place in the body. They self-destruct when they become damaged or too old and become specialised (mature). Cancer cells are different in that they do not stop growing and dividing. The cells keep doubling, forming a tumour growing in size.

Transport systems

Figure 6.1   Simple diffusion.

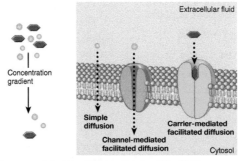

Source: Tortora GJ, Derrickson B. Tortora's Principles of Anatomy and Physiology, 15th edn. Hoboken: Wiley (2017).

Figure 6.2   Channel-mediated facilitated diffusion of potassium ions (K+) through a gated K+ channel.

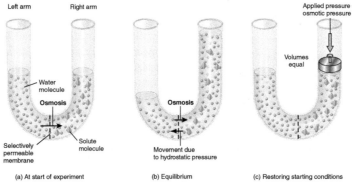

(a) At start of experiment   (b) Equilibrium   (c) Restoring starting conditions

Source: Tortora GJ, Derrickson B. Tortora's Principles of Anatomy and Physiology, 15th edn. Hoboken: Wiley (2017).

Figure 6.3   Osmosis. Water molecules move through the selectively permeable membrane; solute molecules cannot. (a) Water molecules move from the left arm into the right arm, down the water concentration gradient. (b) The volume of water in the left arm has decreased and the volume of solution in the right arm has increased. (c) Pressure applied to the solution in the right arm restores the starting conditions.

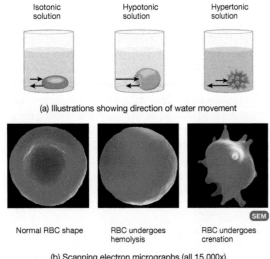

(a) Illustrations showing direction of water movement

Normal RBC shape   RBC undergoes hemolysis   RBC undergoes crenation

(b) Scanning electron micrographs (all 15,000x)

Source: (a) Tortora GJ, Derrickson B. (2017) Tortora's Principles of Anatomy and Physiology, 15th edn. Hoboken: Wiley, (b) David M. Phillips/Science.

Figure 6.4   Tonicity and the red blood cell.

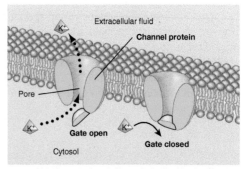

Details of the K⁺ channel

Source: Tortora GJ, Derrickson B. Tortora's Principles of Anatomy and Physiology, 15th edn. Hoboken: Wiley, with permission from John Wiley & Sons (2017).

Anatomy and Physiology for Nursing and Healthcare Students at a Glance, Second Edition. Ian Peate.
© 2022 John Wiley & Sons Ltd. Published 2022 by John Wiley & Sons Ltd.
Companion website: www.wiley.com/go/peate/anatomyandphysiology

Cells perform chemical reactions essential for organism survival. The substances required for these reactions to occur (for example, oxygen and glucose) have to enter the cells and waste products must be removed from the cells. In humans, substances move into and out of cells by osmosis diffusion active transport; plasma membranes are selectively permeable. The cell membrane (see Chapter 5) acts as a gatekeeper, ensuring the cell's cytoplasm remains in place, and will only permit entry to and allow exit from the cell as needed. Three transport systems will be discussed in this chapter: simple diffusion facilitated diffusion and osmosis.

Simple diffusion

This is a passive process in which substances move freely through the lipid bilayer of the plasma membranes of cells; this does not require the help of membrane transport proteins (Figure 6.1). Through the process of simple diffusion, non-polar, hydrophobic molecules move across the lipid bilayer; these include oxygen, carbon dioxide, nitrogen gases; fatty acids, steroids and fat-soluble vitamins. Small, uncharged polar molecules, for example water and urea, also pass through the lipid bilayer by simple diffusion. This type of transport mechanism, occurring through the lipid bilayer, is crucial for the movement of oxygen and carbon dioxide between blood and body cells and also between blood and air occurring within the lungs during breathing. This route is also used for absorption of some nutrients and the excretion of some waste by body cells. While this process occurs spontaneously, the rate of diffusion for different substances is influenced by membrane permeability. It is also influenced by cell properties, the diffusing molecule, temperature of the surrounding solution and the size of the molecule.

Facilitated diffusion

This is a type of diffusion in which molecules are transported across the plasma membrane with the assistance of membrane proteins because the molecules are too polar or highly charged to move through the lipid bilayer by simple diffusion. The molecule to be transported first binds to a receptor site on the carrier protein. The shape of the protein then changes and the molecule is transported into the cell where it is released into the cytoplasm. Once transportation is complete, the protein will then return to its normal shape.

Small non-polar molecules can be easily diffused across the cell membrane but due to the hydrophobic nature of the lipids making up cell membranes, polar molecules, for example water and ions, cannot. A transport protein completely spans the membrane, permitting certain molecules or ions to diffuse across the membrane. Channel proteins, gated channel proteins and carrier proteins are three types of transport proteins that are involved in facilitated diffusion. See Figure 6.2, depicting channel-mediated facilitated diffusion of potassium ions (K+) through a gated K+ channel.

Osmosis

Osmosis refers to the movement of solution from an area of high volume to an area of low volume through a selective permeable membrane. It is a type of diffusion (Figure 6.3). Although osmosis does not utilise energy, it uses kinetic energy. The kinetic energy of an object is the energy that it possesses due to its movement. The movement of water driven by osmosis is known as osmotic flow. The greater the initial difference in solute concentrations, the stronger the osmotic flow.

Those solutions with varying solute concentrations are described as isotonic, hypotonic or hypertonic (Figure 6.4). When a cell is placed in an isotonic solution, there is very little net movement of water in or out of the cell. When placed in a hypotonic solution, water will move into the cell, causing it to swell and burst. However, when the cell is placed in a hypertonic solution, water will move out of the cell, causing it to shrink and die.

Endocytosis and exocytosis

Endocytosis is an energy-using process by which cells absorb molecules (such as proteins) by engulfing them. Endocytosis occurs in three different ways.

1 Phagocytosis: pseudopodia engulf the particle to be imported.
2 Pinocytosis: the cell membrane pinches in to engulf a portion of extracellular fluid containing solutes required by the cell. This process is non-specific; any solutes in the solution will be engulfed.
3 Receptor-mediated endocytosis: this process allows the intake of large quantities of molecules that may not be in high concentration in the extracellular fluid.

Exocytosis is the process by which the cell releases materials to the outside by discharging them as membrane-bound vesicles passing through the cell membrane.

> **Clinical practice point**
> While phagocytosis is an effective defence mechanism, some pathogenic species can escape this process, including *E. coli* and *S. aureus*. Diminished phagocytosis can lead to the development of autoimmune disorders. Phagocytic function is impaired with age.

7 Blood

Figure 7.1 Centrifuged blood.

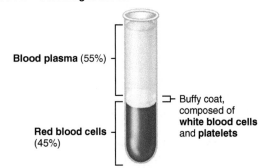

Blood plasma (55%)

Buffy coat, composed of **white blood cells** and **platelets**

Red blood cells (45%)

Appearance of centrifuged blood

Source: Tortora GJ, Derrickson B. Tortora's Principles of Anatomy and Physiology, 15th edn. Hoboken: Wiley, with permission from John Wiley & Sons (2017).

Figure 7.3 Compoments of blood.

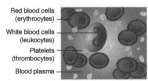

Red blood cells (erythrocytes)

White blood cells (leukocytes)

Platelets (thrombocytes)

Blood plasma

Figure 7.2 Three principal formed components: red blood cells, white blood cells and platelets.

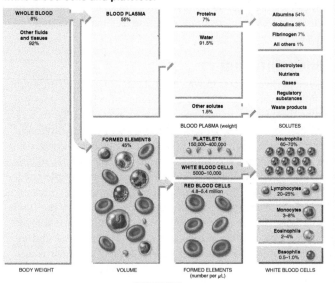

Source: Tortora GJ, Derrickson B. Tortora's Principles of Anatomy and Physiology, 15th edn. Hoboken: Wiley, with permission from John Wiley & Sons (2017).

Figure 7.4 Haemopoiesis.

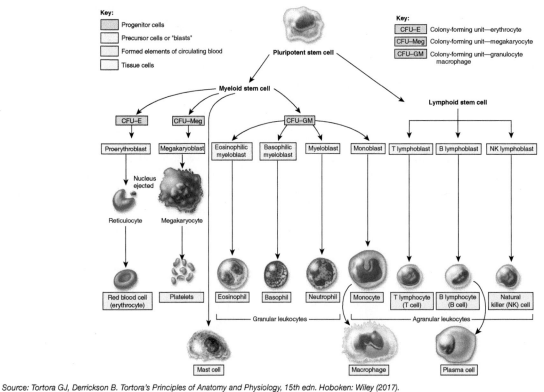

Source: Tortora GJ, Derrickson B. Tortora's Principles of Anatomy and Physiology, 15th edn. Hoboken: Wiley (2017).

Anatomy and Physiology for Nursing and Healthcare Students at a Glance, Second Edition. Ian Peate.
© 2022 John Wiley & Sons Ltd. Published 2022 by John Wiley & Sons Ltd.
Companion website: www.wiley.com/go/peate/anatomyandphysiology

Blood is a liquid connective tissue made up of cells surrounded by a liquid extracellular matrix.

Functions

Transportation

Blood transports oxygen from the lungs to the cells and carbon dioxide from the cells to the lungs to be exhaled. It carries nutrients from the gastrointestinal tract to cells and hormones from endocrine glands to other body cells. Blood is also responsible for the transportation of heat and waste products to several organs for elimination from the body.

Regulation

As the blood circulates, it helps to maintain blood fluid homeostasis by regulating pH through the use of chemicals that convert strong acids or bases into weak ones (known as buffers). It also helps adjust body temperature through the heat-absorbing and coolant properties of the water contained in blood plasma and its fluctuating flow through the skin, via which excess heat can be lost from the blood to the environment. Furthermore, blood osmotic pressure changes the water content of cells.

Protection

As blood clots, it becomes gel-like; after injury, this protects against excessive blood loss from the cardiovascular system. The white blood cells protect against disease as they undertake phagocytosis. Several types of blood proteins, including antibodies, interferons and complement, help to protect against disease in a number of ways.

Blood components

Blood has two components with around 45% formed elements and 55% blood plasma (Figure 7.1). Usually, more than 99% of the formed elements of blood are red blood cells (RBCs). White blood cells (WBCs) and platelets account for less than 1% of the formed elements.

Formed elements of blood

There are three principal formed elements components: red blood cells, white blood cells and platelets (Figure 7.2). Red blood cells or erythrocytes transport oxygen from lungs to body cells, and carbon dioxide from body cells to the lungs. White blood cells or leucocytes offer protection from invading disease-causing organisms and other foreign bodies. There are a number of types of WBCs: neutrophils, basophils, eosinophils, monocytes and lymphocytes. Lymphocytes are further subdivided into B lymphocytes (B cells), T lymphocytes (T cells) and natural killer (NK) cells. Each WBC contributes specifically to the body's defence mechanism. The last formed elements are platelets; these are fragments of cells and have no nucleus. Among other activities, they release chemicals, promoting blood clotting when blood vessels are damaged.

Blood plasma

Plasma is a straw-coloured liquid. Figure 7.3 depicts the composition of blood plasma along with the numbers of the different types of formed elements in blood.

Plasma is about 91.5% water and 8.5% solutes, most of which are proteins. Some of the proteins in blood plasma are found elsewhere in the body; those confined to blood are known as plasma proteins. Certain blood cells develop into cells that produce gamma globulins, an important type of globulin; these are called antibodies or immunoglobulins as they are produced during specific immune responses. Other solutes in plasma include electrolytes, nutrients, regulatory substances, for example enzymes and hormones, gases as well as waste products such as urea, uric acid, creatinine, ammonia and bilirubin.

Development of blood cells

Haemopoiesis describes the process by which the formed elements of blood develop (Figure 7.4). Red bone marrow is the primary centre for haemopoiesis.

Red blood cells are biconcave discs containing oxygen-carrying protein called haemoglobin. The biconcave shape is maintained by a network of proteins called spectrin. This network allows the red blood cells to change shape as they are transported through the blood vessel. Young red blood cells contain a nucleus; this is absent in mature red blood cells, thus increasing the oxygen-carrying capacity of the cell.

Haemoglobin is composed of the protein globin bound to the iron-containing pigment called haem. Each haemoglobin molecule has four atoms of iron, and each atom of iron will transport one molecule of oxygen. There are around 250 million haemoglobin molecules in one RBC and one RBC will transport 1 billion molecules of oxygen

White blood cells circulate for only a short period of their life span; most of their life span is spent migrating through dense and loose connective tissues. All WBCs migrate from the blood vessel by a process known as emigration. Some WBCs are capable of phagocytosis.

Platelets are small blood cells consisting of cytoplasm surrounded by a plasma membrane produced in the bone marrow from megakaryocytes; fragments of megakaryocytes break off to form platelets. They are around 2–4 μm in diameter, they have no nucleus and their life span is approximately 5–9 days. Platelets have a vital role to play in blood loss as they form platelet plugs, sealing the holes in the blood vessels and releasing chemicals that aid blood clotting.

Clinical practice point

A bone marrow sample is obtained in order to diagnose certain blood disorders, such as leukaemia and severe anaemias. This usually involves bone marrow aspiration or a bone marrow biopsy. Both types of samples are usually taken from the iliac crest, although samples can be aspirated from the sternum. The tissue or cell sample is sent for analysis.

8 Inflammation and immunity

Figure 8.1 Types of acquired immunity.

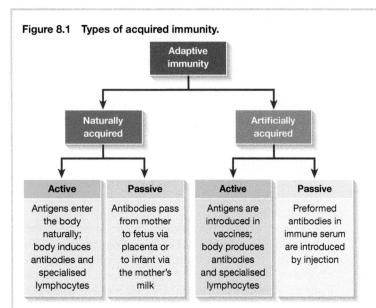

```
                    Adaptive
                    immunity
          ┌────────────┴────────────┐
     Naturally                  Artificially
     acquired                     acquired
    ┌────┴────┐              ┌────────┴────────┐
 Active    Passive        Active           Passive
```

Active	Passive	Active	Passive
Antigens enter the body naturally; body induces antibodies and specialised lymphocytes	Antibodies pass from mother to fetus via placenta or to infant via the mother's milk	Antigens are introduced in vaccines; body produces antibodies and specialised lymphocytes	Preformed antibodies in immune serum are introduced by injection

Table 8.1 Types of antibodies.

Type of antibody	Functions
IgA	Found in breast milk, mucous, saliva and tears prevents antigens from crossing epithelial membranes and invading the deeper tissues
IgD	Produced by B cells and is displayed on their surface. Antigens bind to active B cells here
IgE	The least common antibody. Found bound to tissue cell membranes particularly eosinophils
IgG	The most common and largest antibody. Attacks various pathogens, crossing the placenta to protect the fetus
IgM	Produced in large quantities, is the primary response and a powerful activator of complement

Figure 8.2 The cells of the immune system.

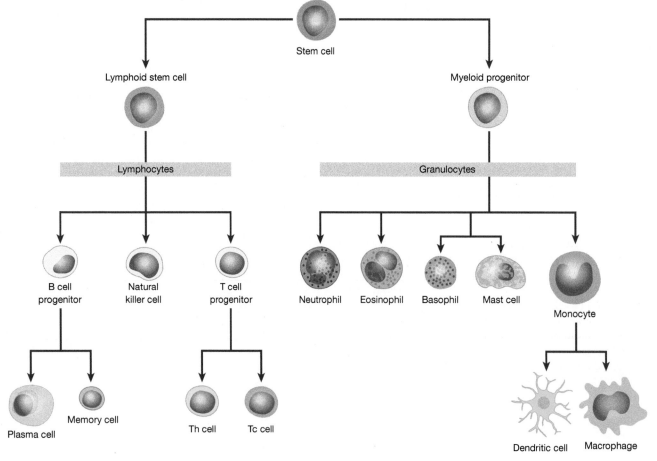

Stem cell

Lymphoid stem cell

Myeloid progenitor

Lymphocytes

Granulocytes

B cell progenitor

Natural killer cell

T cell progenitor

Neutrophil

Eosinophil

Basophil

Mast cell

Monocyte

Plasma cell

Memory cell

Th cell

Tc cell

Dendritic cell

Macrophage

Anatomy and Physiology for Nursing and Healthcare Students at a Glance, Second Edition. Ian Peate.
© 2022 John Wiley & Sons Ltd. Published 2022 by John Wiley & Sons Ltd.
Companion website: www.wiley.com/go/peate/anatomyandphysiology

Inflammation is one of the key processes stimulating the immune system. The immune response is how the body recognises and defends itself against bacteria, viruses and substances seen as foreign and potentially harmful.

Immunity

Immunity provides the opportunity to address disease and harm through defence mechanisms. When there is absence of resistance, this is known as susceptibility. There are two broad types of immunity: innate and aquired (also called adaptive).

Innate immunity

Innate (non-specific) immunity refers to defences present at birth. Innate immunity does not involve specific recognition of a microbe, it acts against all microbes in the same way (hence non-specific). Innate immune responses are the body's early warning system and are intended to prevent microbes from entering the body and to help with the elimination of those that do enter the body.

The first line of defence against pathogens is the skin and mucous membranes of the body. These offer physical and chemical barriers that prevent pathogens and foreign substances gaining entry to the body and bringing about disease. When pathogens penetrate the physical and chemical barriers of the skin and mucous membranes, a second line of defence is encountered: internal antimicrobial substances, phagocytes, natural killer cells, inflammation and fever.

Acquired immunity

This is also known as specific immunity as it only responds to known, specific organisms that we have previously encountered (have previously infected us). The acquired immunity system remembers when a particular immunological threat has been met and overcome, recalling how to defeat it and mobilise the immune system to counter that threat (immunological memory). The acquired immune system is based upon lymphocytes, closely associated with the lymphatic system.

The primary response (exposure for the first time) produces a slow and delayed rise in antibody levels. The delay is associated with activation of the T lymphocyte system that stimulates B lymphocyte separation.

The secondary response occurs on subsequent exposure to the same antigen; the response in this case is much faster as the memory B lymphocytes generated after the first infection divide and separate at a much faster rate, and antibody production occurs almost immediately (see Table 8.1 for the five types of antibody).

Natural and artificially acquired immunity

Immunity can be acquired naturally or artificially; both can be active or passive (Figure 8.1).

When active immunity occurs, this indicates that the person has made a response to an antigen, leading to the production of their own antibodies with activation of lymphocytes; the memory cells offer long-lasting resistance.

Passive immunity occurs when the individual has been given antibodies. This type of immunity is fairly short-acting as the antibodies eventually break down.

Inflammation

When tissue damage occurs, a number of proteins are activated, the catalyst for the immune response. This response is non-specific, attacking any and all foreign invaders in an attempt to rid the body of microbes, toxins or other foreign matter, aiming to prevent their spread to other tissues, preparing the site for tissue repair and restoring tissue homeostasis.

Cells of the immune system find and destroy damaged cells and foreign tissues, while recognising and preserving host cells (Figure 8.2). Four phases occur in the inflammatory response: redness, swelling, heat and pain.

When injury occurs, almost instantaneously the damaged cells instigate a number of events: vasodilation, release of messenger molecules, initiation of complement, extravasation of vascular components, phagocytosis and pain.

Injured mast cells release histamine, arterioles dilate and venules constrict, encouraging an increase in blood flow. The main mechanisms associated with vasodilation are the production of bradykinin (a vasodilator; also causes pain) and release of arachidonic acid, a fatty acid, a precursor to prostaglandins. Prostaglandins (vasodilators) can increase pain. Histamine from the degranulated mast cells enlarges pore size between capillary cells and proteins and other micromolecules move into interstitial spaces. Nitric oxide is released, causing further vasodilation; the presence of macrophages releases large quantities of nitric oxide.

Cells close to the injury release chemokines. The concentration of chemokines is greatest immediately surrounding the infection; high levels of chemokines attract phagocytic white blood cells, including neutrophils.

As chemokine concentration increases, the phagocytes leave the capillary, entering the site of infection; macrophages arrive around 24 hours later. Phagocytes engulf and destroy the pathogens present, recognising them as non-self matter. The key molecule released is interleukin 1 which attracts neutrophils and macrophages to the site of injury, helping to clear away debris from the injured area.

Clinical practice point

Nurses and other health and social care professionals have a key role to play in promoting immunisation. This includes the administration of those vaccinations that are included in the childhood immunisation programme as well as those that are recommended for adults. Health and care professionals are an important and trusted source of advice with regard to vaccination. Discussion with parents and the public is time well spent and people welcome having the opportunity to ask questions and seek advice from reliable sources.

9 Tissues

Figure 9.1 Levels of organisation.

Atom → Molecule or compound → Organelle → Cell → Tissue → Organ → Organ system → Organism

Figure 9.2 Types of cells.

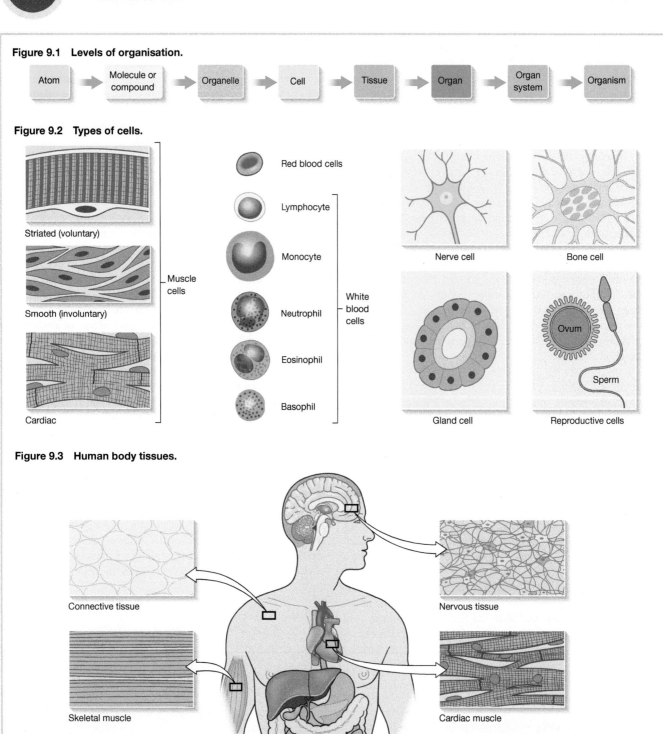

Striated (voluntary)
Smooth (involuntary)
Cardiac
} Muscle cells

Red blood cells
Lymphocyte
Monocyte
Neutrophil
Eosinophil
Basophil
} White blood cells

Nerve cell
Bone cell
Gland cell
Ovum / Sperm — Reproductive cells

Figure 9.3 Human body tissues.

Connective tissue
Skeletal muscle
Epithelial tissue
Nervous tissue
Cardiac muscle
Smooth muscle

Anatomy and Physiology for Nursing and Healthcare Students at a Glance, Second Edition. Ian Peate.
© 2022 John Wiley & Sons Ltd. Published 2022 by John Wiley & Sons Ltd.
Companion website: www.wiley.com/go/peate/anatomyandphysiology

There are many types of cells in the body, organised into four distinct categories of tissues: epithelial, connective, nervous and muscle. Within these four categories, there are several subdivisions. Each of these categories is characterised by specific functions, contributing to the overall health and maintenance of the body. Generally, tissue types are composed of similar cells carrying out associated functions; for example, the epidermis of the face and the buccal mucosa (lining of the mouth) are the same tissue type with related functions but their appearance is very different to the naked eye. Blood and bone look very different yet both are classified in the same tissue type. Tissues, made up of large numbers of cells, are classified according to their size, shape and functions (Figures 9.1–9.3).

Epithelial tissue

Epithelial tissue is located in the covering of external and internal surfaces of the body, and the hollow organs and tubes; it is also found in the glands. The overall function of the epithelium is to offer protection and impermeability (or selective permeability) to the covered structure. Cells are closely packed and the matrix (the intracellular substance) is minimal. Usually there is a basement membrane on which the cells lie. The epithelial tissue can be simple (a single layer of cells); subdivided into squamous epithelium (forms the lining of the heart, blood vessels, lymph vessels, alveoli of the lungs, lining of the collecting ducts of the nephrons); or stratified where there are several layers of tissue, composed of several layers of these cells. Keratinised stratified epithelium is found on dry surfaces exposed to wear and tear such as the skin, hair and nails. Non-keratinised epithelium protects those moist surfaces that are subjected to wear and tear, such as the conjunctiva, the linings of the mouth and the vagina. The urinary bladder is lined with transitional epithelium which permits the bladder to stretch as it fills.

Nervous tissue

This is made up of neurons and glial cells. Its function is to receive and transmit neural impulses (reception and transmission of information). Two types of tissue are found in the nervous system: excitable cells (the neurons – initiate, receive, conduct and transmit information) and non-excitable cells (the glial cells – supporting the neurons). A neuron is made up of two major parts: the cell body, containing the neuron's nucleus, and cytoplasm and other organelles. Nerve processes are 'finger-like' projections arising from the cell body and can conduct and transmit signals. There are two types: axons carrying signals away from the cell body and dendrites carrying signals toward the cell body. Neurons usually have one axon (this can be branched). Axons normally terminate at a synapse through which the signal is sent to the next cell, typically through a dendrite.

Connective tissue

There are many kinds of connective tissue and it is the most abundant type of tissue; connective tissue is typically used to fill empty spaces between other body tissues. The cells of connective tissue secrete substances that compose extracellular material, such as collagen and elastic fibres, creating a considerable spacing between these cells. Other important biological features include substance transportation, protection of the organism and insulation. Connective tissue (excluding blood) is found in organs supporting specialised tissues.

The matrix of areolar connective tissue is semi-solid, containing adipocytes, mast cells and macrophages. Where there is a need to provide elasticity and tensile strength, areola tissue is present, for example under the skin, between muscles and in the alimentary canal. Adipose tissue supports the kidneys, brain and eyes and is related to energy intake and expenditure. Lymphoid tissue contains reticular cells and white blood cells, and is located in lymph tissue in the lymph nodes and lymphatic organs. Dense connective tissue (fibrous tissue composed of closely packed collagen fibres with little matrix) is found in ligaments, periosteum, muscle fascia and tendons. Blood is a fluid connective tissue. Cartilage is found as hyaline cartilage on the ends of the bones that form joints, the costal cartilage attaching the ribs to the sternum, and in the trachea, larynx and bronchi. Bone cells are surrounded by a matrix of collagen fibres with added strength provided by calcium and phosphate.

Muscle tissue

Muscle tissues are made of cells that permit contractions, generating movement. The function of muscle tissue is to pull bones (skeletal striated muscle), to contract and move viscera and vessels (smooth muscle), and make the heart beat (cardiac striated muscle). Muscle is involved each time we move, breathe, ingest food or urinate. The muscle cells comprise internal structures, called sarcomeres, in which myosin and actin molecules work to create contraction and movement.

There are three kinds of muscle in the body: skeletal, cardiac and smooth muscle. Skeletal muscle (striated muscle) is a voluntary muscle. Cells in skeletal muscle are long and thin with multiple nuclei. Cardiac muscle is only found in the heart, with the muscle fibres interlocking with each other to ensure that as one aspect of the muscle is stimulated, all other stimulated fibres contract sequentially. Cardiac muscle is not under voluntary control; the special cells of the sinoatrial node are responsible for sending out impulses resulting in cardiac contraction. Smooth muscle is involuntary, held together by connective tissue with bands of elastic protein wrapped around them. Smooth muscle is seen in the walls of hollow structures and vessels: blood vessels, ureters, urinary bladder, parts of the respiratory tract, ducts and glands of the alimentary tract.

Clinical practice point

A disruption of the structure of tissue is a sign of injury or disease. These changes can be detected through histology, which is the microscopic study of tissue appearance, organisation and function. When learning to care for people safely and effectively, this requires the nurse to appreciate the microscopic and macroscopic aspects of the human. Exploring how the body's tissues function permits you to appreciate what can happen when cells, tissues and organ systems fail.

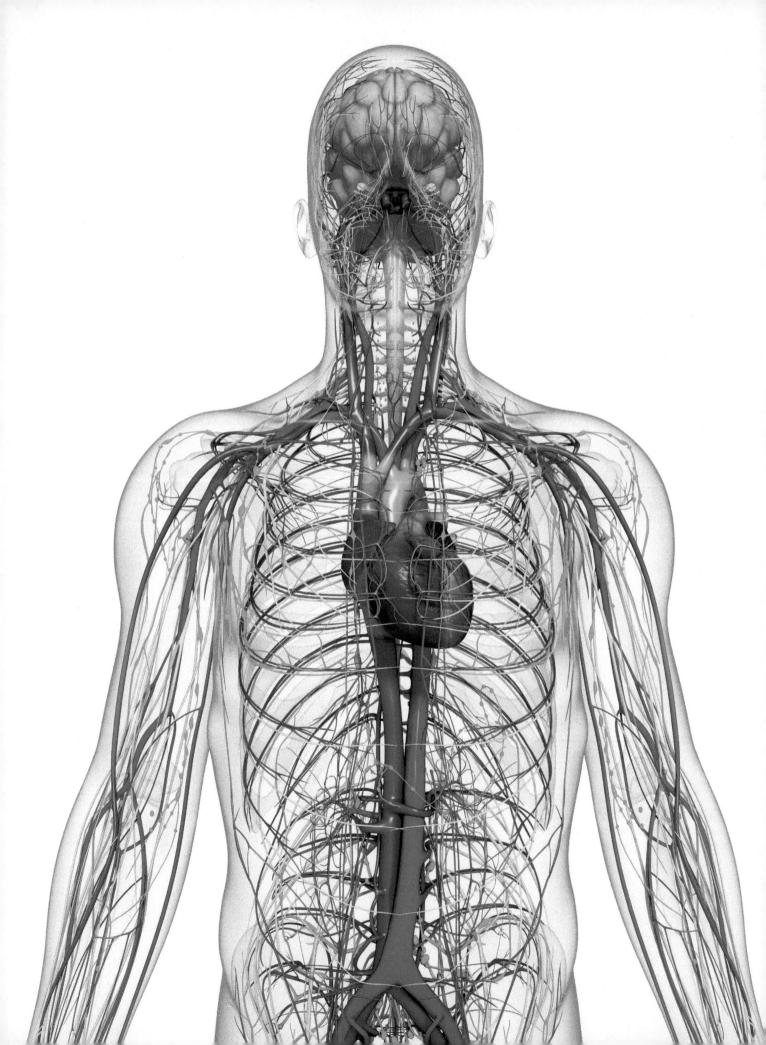

The nervous system

Part 2

Chapters

10 The brain and nerves

Figure 10.1   The brain.

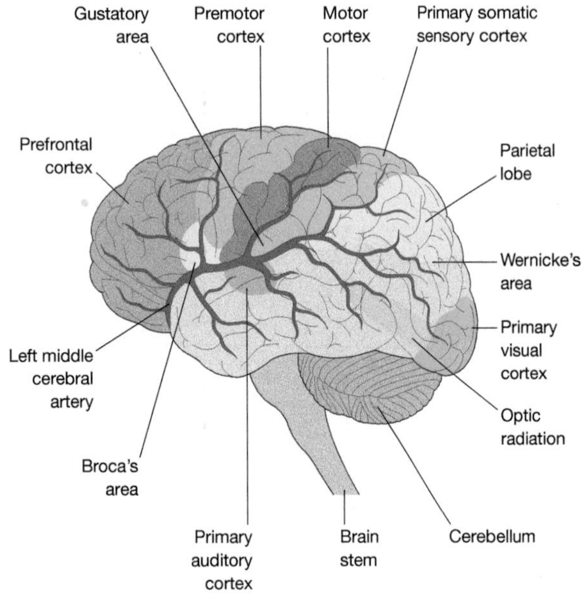

- Gustatory area
- Premotor cortex
- Motor cortex
- Primary somatic sensory cortex
- Prefrontal cortex
- Parietal lobe
- Wernicke's area
- Primary visual cortex
- Left middle cerebral artery
- Optic radiation
- Broca's area
- Primary auditory cortex
- Brain stem
- Cerebellum

Figure 10.3   The neuron.

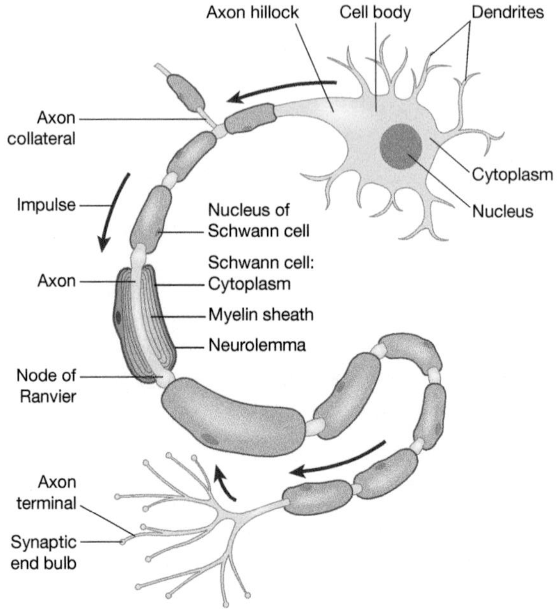

- Axon hillock
- Cell body
- Dendrites
- Axon collateral
- Cytoplasm
- Nucleus
- Impulse
- Nucleus of Schwann cell
- Schwann cell: Cytoplasm
- Axon
- Myelin sheath
- Neurolemma
- Node of Ranvier
- Axon terminal
- Synaptic end bulb

Source: Peate I, Wild K & Nair M (eds). Nursing Practice: Knowledge and Care (2014).

Figure 10.2   The meninges.

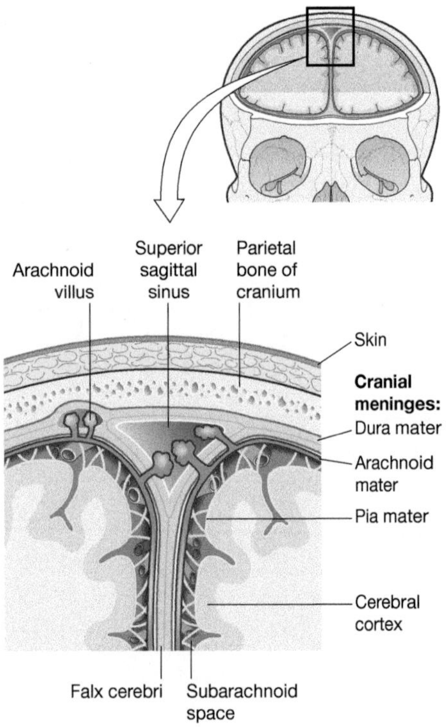

- Arachnoid villus
- Superior sagittal sinus
- Parietal bone of cranium
- Skin
- **Cranial meninges:**
- Dura mater
- Arachnoid mater
- Pia mater
- Cerebral cortex
- Falx cerebri
- Subarachnoid space

Source: Peate I, Wild K & Nair M (eds). Nursing Practice: Knowledge and Care (2014).

Figure 10.4   The cranial nerves.

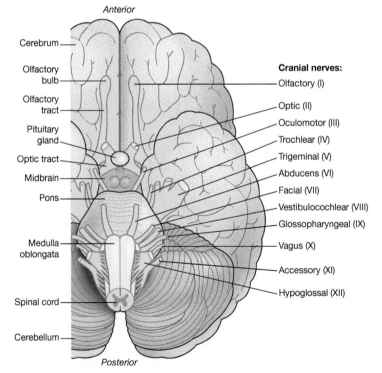

- Anterior
- Cerebrum
- Olfactory bulb
- Olfactory tract
- Pituitary gland
- Optic tract
- Midbrain
- Pons
- Medulla oblongata
- Spinal cord
- Cerebellum
- Posterior

Cranial nerves:
- Olfactory (I)
- Optic (II)
- Oculomotor (III)
- Trochlear (IV)
- Trigeminal (V)
- Abducens (VI)
- Facial (VII)
- Vestibulocochlear (VIII)
- Glossopharyngeal (IX)
- Vagus (X)
- Accessory (XI)
- Hypoglossal (XII)

Source: Peate I, Wild K & Nair M (eds). Nursing Practice: Knowledge and Care (2014).

Anatomy and Physiology for Nursing and Healthcare Students at a Glance, Second Edition. Ian Peate.
© 2022 John Wiley & Sons Ltd. Published 2022 by John Wiley & Sons Ltd.
Companion website: www.wiley.com/go/peate/anatomyandphysiology

The brain

The brain is one of the largest and most complex organs in the body. It is responsible for the integration of sensory information (for example, it interprets the senses); it also directs motor responses (it is the initiator of body movement and controller of behaviour) and is the centre of learning.

The brain weighs around 1400 grams. It is protected inside a bony shell (the cranium or skull) and washed by protective fluid (cerebrospinal fluid). It is the source of all those qualities that define us as humans (Figure 10.1).

The brain receives 15% of the cardiac output. It has a system of autoregulation making sure that its blood supply is constant regardless of positional changes. Most of the expansion comes from the cerebral cortex, a convoluted layer of neural tissue covering the surface. The frontal lobes are particularly expanded and are involved in executive functions, such as self-control, planning, reasoning and abstract thought.

The meninges

As nervous tissue can be easily damaged by pressure, it needs to be protected. The hair, skin and bone provide an outer layer of protection. Closest to the nervous tissue are the meninges which cover the delicate nervous tissue. They also protect the blood vessels that serve nervous tissue and they contain cerebrospinal fluid. The meninges are made up of three connective tissue layers: dura, arachnoid and pia maters (Figure 10.2).

The cerebrospinal fluid

The cerebrospinal fluid (CSF) is produced by the choroid plexus located within the ventricles of the brain. Approximately 150 mL of CSF circulates around the brain, in the ventricles and around the spinal cord. Every 8 hours the CSF is replaced. The CSF provides a cushion to the brain to protect it from damage, it maintains a uniform pressure between the brain and spinal cord, and plays a small role in fluid and waste exchange between the brain and spinal cord.

The neuron

The functional unit of the brain is the neuron or nerve cell (Figure 10.3). A neuron has a number of features in common with other cells, including a nucleus and mitochondria. However, because of its key role, it is well protected with some specialist modifications.

Neurons are composed of an axon, dendrites and a cell body. Their function is to transmit nerve impulses. Nerve impulses only ever travel in one direction: from the receptive area – the dendrites – to the cell body and down the length of the axon.

Axon

Each neuron has only one axon, but the axon can branch to form an axon collateral (see Figure 10.3). The axon will also branch at its end into several axon terminals. The axon length may vary quite significantly, from very short to 100 cm long. The axon is much thicker and longer than the dendrites of a neuron. Larger neurons have a noticeably expanded region at the start of the axon, known as the axon hillock, which is the site of summation for incoming information. At any given moment, the combined influence of all axons that conduct impulses to a given neuron determines whether or not an action potential will be initiated at the axon hillock and disseminated along the axon.

Dendrites

Dendrites are the short branching processes that receive information. Generally, dendrites are very thin appendages, becoming narrower as they extend further away from the cell body (see Figure 10.3). Dendritic spines are short outgrowths that further increase the receptive surface area of a neuron. The surface of dendrite branches is covered with junctions designed for the reception of incoming information. Their branching processes provide a large surface area for this function. In sensory neurons, the dendrites frequently form part of the sensory receptors and in motor neurons they can be part of the synapse between one neuron and the next.

Cell body

The cell body (soma) is the central part of the neuron. It contains the nucleus of the cell and as such it is where most protein synthesis occurs. The nucleus ranges from 3 to 18 micrometers in diameter. Most of the neuron cell bodies (see Figure 10.3) are found inside the central nervous system, forming the grey matter. When there are clusters of cell bodies grouped together in the central nervous system, they are known as nuclei. Cell bodies found in the peripheral nervous system are called ganglia.

Myelin sheath

Oligodendrocytes and Schwann cells form the myelin sheaths that insulate axons in the central and peripheral nervous systems, respectively. Peripheral nerve axons and long or large axons are covered in a myelin sheath (see Figure 10.3). Myelin is a fatty material that protects the neuron as well as electrically insulating it, which speeds up impulse transmission. Schwann cells, wrapped in layers around the neuron within the peripheral nervous system, form the myelin sheath. The outermost part of the Schwann cell is its plasma membrane, called the neurilemma. There is a regular gap (about 1 μm) between adjacent Schwann cells called the nodes of Ranvier. Collateral axons can occur at the node. Some nerve fibres are unmyelinated and nerve impulse transmission in these fibres is significantly slower.

Cranial nerves

There are 12 pairs of cranial nerves emerging from the brain and supplying various structures, most of which are associated with the head and neck (Figure 10.4). The cranial nerves vary in their functions; some are sensory nerves, containing only sensory fibres, some are motor nerves, containing only motor fibres, and some are mixed nerves, containing both sensory and motor fibres.

Clinical practice point

Multiple sclerosis is a disease that affects the central nervous system. The immune system attacks the myelin, the protective layer around nerve fibres, and causes inflammation and lesions. This makes it difficult for the brain to send signals to the rest of the body. The most common symptoms of multiple sclerosis include eye problems, numbness or tingling feelings, fatigue and pain. The symptoms can come and go and may change over time. They can be mild or more severe. The healthcare provider must ensure an individual assessment of needs is carried out and individual care plans are implemented and evaluated.

11 The structures of the brain

Figure 11.1   The cerebrum.

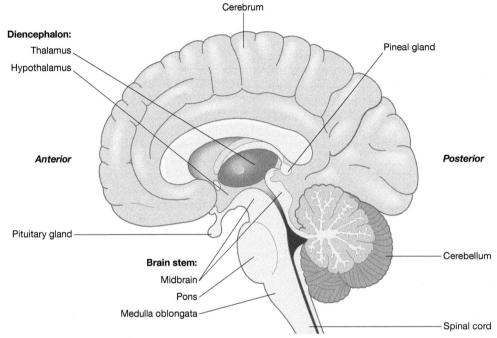

Cerebrum

Diencephalon:
Thalamus
Hypothalamus

Pineal gland

Anterior

Posterior

Pituitary gland

Brain stem:
Midbrain
Pons
Medulla oblongata

Cerebellum

Spinal cord

Source: Peate I, Wild K & Nair M (eds). Nursing Practice: Knowledge and Care (2014).

Figure 11.2   The cerebellum.

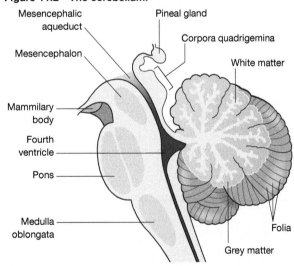

Mesencephalic aqueduct
Mesencephalon
Mammilary body
Fourth ventricle
Pons
Medulla oblongata

Pineal gland
Corpora quadrigemina
White matter
Folia
Grey matter

Figure 11.3   The limbic system.

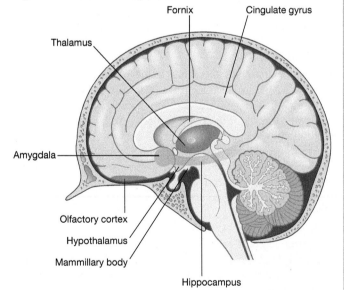

Fornix
Cingulate gyrus
Thalamus
Amygdala
Olfactory cortex
Hypothalamus
Mammillary body
Hippocampus

The four major regions of the brain are:
- the cerebrum
- the diencephalon
- the brainstem
- the cerebellum.

Cerebrum

The cerebrum, also known as the telencephalon, is the largest and most highly developed part of the brain. It covers around two-thirds of the brain mass and lies over and around most of the structures of the brain (Figure 11.1). The cerebrum sits on top of the brainstem, with the cerebellum underneath the rear portion.

The cerebrum of an adult is divided into two large hemispheres (the left and right hemispheres). The surfaces of the cerebral hemispheres are highly folded and covered by a superficial layer of grey matter known as the cerebral cortex. The functions of the cerebrum include regulation of muscle contraction, memory storage and processing, production of speech, interpretation of taste, sound and memory for storage and processing.

Diencephalon

The diencephalon provides a functional link between the cerebral hemispheres and the rest of the central nervous system (CNS). It contains three paired structures: the thalamus, hypothalamus and epithalamus. Each component of the diencephalon has specialised functions that are integral to life.

Thalamus

The thalamus acts as a relay station for sensory impulses going to the cerebral cortex for integration and motor impulses entering and leaving the cerebral hemispheres. It also plays a role in memory.

Hypothalamus

The hypothalamus is closely associated with the pituitary gland and produces two hormones: antidiuretic hormone (ADH) and oxytocin. It is also the chief autonomic integration centre and is part of the limbic system, which is the emotional brain.

Epithalamus

The epithalamus is a small structure that is linked to the pineal gland, which secretes the hormone melatonin responsible for sleep/wake cycles.

Brainstem

The brainstem regulates vital cardiac and respiratory functions and acts as a vehicle for sensory information.

The structures that form the brainstem are involved in a range of activities that are essential for life. The brainstem is associated with the cranial nerves. The structures of the brainstem include the midbrain, pons and medulla oblongata (see Figure 11.1).

Midbrain

The midbrain contains nuclei that deal with auditory and visual information and reflexes. It also maintains consciousness and provides a conduction pathway connecting the cerebrum with the lower brain structures and spinal cord.

Pons

The pons connects and communicates with the cerebellum. It works with the medulla oblongata to control the depth and rate of respiration and contains nuclei that function in visceral and somatic motor control.

Medulla oblongata

The medulla oblongata is a relay station for sensory nerves going to the cerebrum. The medulla contains autonomic centres such as the cardiac centre, respiratory centre, vasomotor centre and coughing, sneezing and vomiting centres. The medulla is also the site of decussation of the pyramidal tract; this means that the right side of the body is controlled by the left cerebral hemisphere and vice versa.

Cerebellum

The second largest structure of the brain (Figure 11.2), partially hidden by the cerebral hemispheres, is the cerebellum. The cerebellum is responsible for the co-ordination of voluntary muscle movement, motor learning, cognitive functions and balance and posture. It ensures that muscle movements are smooth, co-ordinated and precise. Motor commands are not initiated in the cerebellum; the cerebellum modifies the motor commands of the descending pathways to ensure that movements are more adaptive and accurate. Even though the cerebellum accounts for approximately 10% of the brain's volume, it contains over 50% of the total number of neurons in the brain.

Limbic system

The limbic system is a complex set of brain structures located on both sides of the thalamus, under the cerebrum. The limbic system includes the hippocampus, amygdala, anterior thalamic nuclei, septum, habenula, limbic cortex and fornix. It supports a variety of functions, including emotion, behaviour, motivation, long-term memory and olfaction. The limbic system acts on the endocrine and autonomic nervous systems (Figure 11.3).

Ventricles of the brain

These are a series of interconnected, fluid-filled cavities that lie within the brain, a communicating network filled with cerebrospinal fluid (CSF) and located within the brain parenchyma. The ventricular system is composed of two lateral ventricles, the third ventricle, the cerebral aqueduct, and the fourth ventricle. The choroid plexuses located in the ventricles produce CSF, filling the ventricles and subarachnoid space, following a cycle of constant production and reabsorption.

Cerebrospinal fluid

Cerebrospinal fluid is a clear body fluid occupying the subarachnoid space and the brain ventricular system around and inside the brain and spinal cord. It acts as a cushion or buffer for the cortex, providing basic mechanical and immunological protection to the brain inside the skull. It is produced by modified ependymal cells of the choroid plexus found in all components of the ventricular system except for the cerebral aqueduct and the posterior and anterior horns of the lateral ventricles. CSF flows from the lateral ventricle to the third ventricle through the interventricular foramen (also called the foramen of Monro). The third ventricle and fourth ventricle are connected to each other by the cerebral aqueduct (also called the aqueduct of Sylvius). CSF then flows into the subarachnoid space through the foramina of Luschka (there are two of these) and the foramen of Magendie (only one of these).

There is approximately 150 mL of CSF circulating around the brain, in the ventricles and around the spinal cord. The CSF is replaced every 8 hours. Absorption of the CSF into the bloodstream takes place in the superior sagittal sinus through structures called arachnoid villi. When the CSF pressure is greater than the venous pressure, CSF will flow into the bloodstream. However, the arachnoid villi act as 'one-way valves': if the CSF pressure is less than the venous pressure, the arachnoid villi will *not* let blood pass into the ventricular system.

> **Clinical practice point**
>
> Due to the brain's many important roles, damage to any of its lobes from injuries, illnesses or chronic conditions such as brain tumour can cause major losses in brain function. A space-occupying lesion of the brain is usually due to malignancy but it can be caused by other pathologies such as an abscess or haematoma. The effect of a tumour may be local, due to focal brain damage, and the presentation can provide an indication of the location of the lesion but not its cause. There may be more general symptoms related to raised intracranial pressure or seizures, behavioural changes or false localising signs. While large lesions in some regions, for example the frontal lobe, may be relatively silent, a small lesion in the dominant hemisphere may impact severely on speech, for example.

12 The spinal cord

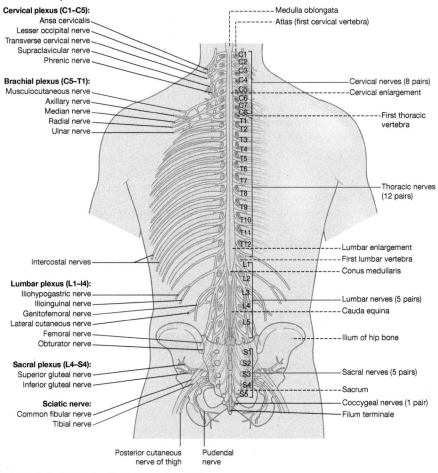

Figure 12.1 Spinal cord and spinal nerves.

Cervical plexus (C1–C5):
Ansa cervicalis
Lesser occipital nerve
Transverse cervical nerve
Supraclavicular nerve
Phrenic nerve

Brachial plexus (C5–T1):
Musculocutaneous nerve
Axillary nerve
Median nerve
Radial nerve
Ulnar nerve

Intercostal nerves

Lumbar plexus (L1–I4):
Iliohypogastric nerve
Ilioinguinal nerve
Genitofemoral nerve
Lateral cutaneous nerve
Femoral nerve
Obturator nerve

Sacral plexus (L4–S4):
Superior gluteal nerve
Inferior gluteal nerve

Sciatic nerve:
Common fibular nerve
Tibial nerve

Posterior cutaneous nerve of thigh
Pudendal nerve

Medulla oblongata
Atlas (first cervical vertebra)
Cervical nerves (8 pairs)
Cervical enlargement
First thoracic vertebra
Thoracic nerves (12 pairs)
Lumbar enlargement
First lumbar vertebra
Conus medullaris
Lumbar nerves (5 pairs)
Cauda equina
Ilium of hip bone
Sacral nerves (5 pairs)
Sacrum
Coccygeal nerves (1 pair)
Filum terminale

Source: Peate I, Wild K & Nair M (eds). Nursing Practice: Knowledge and Care (2014).

Figure 12.2 The meninges.

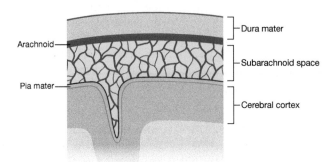

Arachnoid
Pia mater

Dura mater
Subarachnoid space
Cerebral cortex

Anatomy and Physiology for Nursing and Healthcare Students at a Glance, Second Edition. Ian Peate.
© 2022 John Wiley & Sons Ltd. Published 2022 by John Wiley & Sons Ltd.
Companion website: www.wiley.com/go/peate/anatomyandphysiology

The spinal cord is approximately 45 cm in length and 14 mm in width (Figure 12.1). The spinal cord extends from the foramen magnum at the base of the skull to the level of the first lumbar vertebra. The cord is continuous with the medulla oblongata at the foramen magnum. The spinal cord, like the brain, is surrounded by bone, meninges and CSF. There are two layers: an outer layer of white matter and an inner layer of grey matter, which surrounds a small central canal. The spinal cord is enclosed within the vertebral canal forming a protective ring of bone around the cord. Other protective coverings include the spinal meninges, which are three layers of connective tissue which extend around the spinal cord. The spinal meninges consist of the pia mater (inner layer), arachnoid mater (middle layer) and dura mater (the outermost layer which consists of a dense, irregular connective tissue).

Pia mater

The pia mater, or pia, is the delicate innermost layer of the meninges, the membranes surrounding the brain and spinal cord (Figure 12.2). The pia mater is the thin, translucent, mesh-like meningeal envelope, spanning nearly the entire surface of the brain. It is firmly adhered to the surface of the brain and loosely connected to the arachnoid layer. The pia mater covers and protects the central nervous system (CNS), protects the blood vessels and encloses the venous sinuses near the CNS, contains the cerebrospinal fluid (CSF) and forms partitions within the skull.

Arachnoid mater

The arachnoid mater is the protective membrane covering the brain and spinal cord (see Figure 12.2). It includes a simple squamous epithelium known as the arachnoid membrane and the arachnoid trabeculae which is a network of collagen elastic fibres that extend between the arachnoid membrane and the outer surface of the pia mater.

Dura mater

This thin membrane is the outermost of the three layers of the meninges, surrounding the brain and spinal cord (see Figure 12.2). The dura mater has a number of functions and layers. It is a sac that envelops the arachnoid mater, surrounding and supporting the dural sinuses, and carries blood from the brain toward the heart.

Spinal cord sections

The spinal cord is divided into 31 different segments. At each segment, right and left pairs of spinal nerves (mixed: sensory and motor) form. Six to eight motor nerve rootlets branch out of right and left ventrolateral sulci in a very orderly manner. Nerve rootlets combine to form nerve roots.

Each segment of the spinal cord is associated with a pair of ganglia, called dorsal root ganglia, located just outside the spinal cord. The ganglia contain cell bodies of sensory neurons. Axons of these sensory neurons travel into the spinal cord via the dorsal roots.

The spinal cord is supplied with blood by three arteries that run along its length, starting in the brain, and many arteries that approach it through the sides of the spinal column. The three longitudinal arteries are called the anterior spinal artery and the right and left posterior spinal arteries. These travel in the subarachnoid space and send branches into the spinal cord.

Functions of the spinal cord

The spinal cord offers a means of communication between the brain and the peripheral nerves that leave the spinal cord. It has two major functions in maintaining homeostasis.

- The tracts of white matter of the spinal cord carry sensory impulses to the brain and motor impulses from the brain to the skeletal muscles and other effector muscles.
- The grey matter, located in the centre of the cord, is shaped like a butterfly and consists of cell bodies of interneurons and motor neurons. The grey matter is a site for integration of reflexes, which is a rapid, involuntary action in relation to a particular stimulus.

Reflex actions

The spinal cord controls some other important functions, for example reflex actions. For reflex actions, the spinal cord does not need any assistance from the brain. Reflex actions are automatic, unlearned, involuntary and inborn responses. Therefore, these actions are sudden in nature and have the purpose of protecting the individual from sudden danger. For example, if someone were to throw a stone at you, you would automatically move your body to avoid the danger of being hurt.

The path through which reflex action is conducted is called the 'reflex arc', which involves (1) receptor, (2) afferent neuron, (3) spinal cord, (4) interneuron, (5) efferent neuron, and (6) muscles or gland.

Spinal nerves

There are 31 pairs of spinal nerves that are attached to the spinal cord which are named and numbered according to the region and level of the vertebral column from which they emerge. Each nerve innervates a group of muscles (myotome) and an area of skin (dermatome) and most also innervate some of the thoracic and abdominal organs.

The spinal nerves provide the paths of communication between the spinal cord and specific regions of the body as they connect the CNS to sensory receptors, muscles and glands in all parts of the body. A typical spinal nerve has two connections to the spinal cord: a posterior root and an anterior root which unite to form a spinal nerve at the intervertebral foramen. A spinal nerve is an example of a mixed nerve as it contains both sensory (posterior root) and motor (anterior root) fibres.

Clinical practice point

Cauda equina syndrome occurs when the cauda equina nerves are compressed. Compression can occur for a number of reasons, including but not limited to degenerative changes in the spine, a slipped disc, a tumour or spinal abscess. When the nerves are compressed, this typically results in what are commonly referred to as 'red flag' symptoms. Cauda equina syndrome is a medical emergency and if decompression surgery is delayed it can result in lifelong disability. The red flag symptoms to be alert to are lower back pain, pain in one or both legs (often radiates down the leg(s)), leg weakness or altered sensation in one or both legs, foot drop, reduced sensation around the 'saddle' area, such as the groin, genitals, anus and buttocks, loss of or altered control of bladder and bowel function and altered sexual sensation or function.

13 The blood supply

Figure 13.1   The circle of Willis.

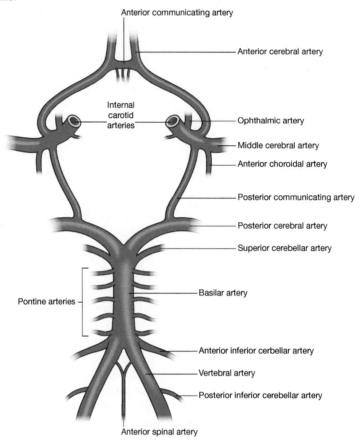

- Anterior communicating artery
- Anterior cerebral artery
- Internal carotid arteries
- Ophthalmic artery
- Middle cerebral artery
- Anterior choroidal artery
- Posterior communicating artery
- Posterior cerebral artery
- Superior cerebellar artery
- Pontine arteries
- Basilar artery
- Anterior inferior cerbellar artery
- Vertebral artery
- Posterior inferior cerebellar artery
- Anterior spinal artery

Figure 13.2   The blood–brain barrier.

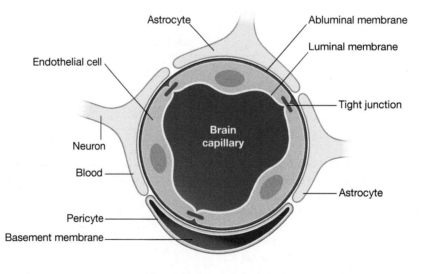

- Astrocyte
- Abluminal membrane
- Luminal membrane
- Endothelial cell
- Tight junction
- Neuron
- Brain capillary
- Blood
- Astrocyte
- Pericyte
- Basement membrane

Anatomy and Physiology for Nursing and Healthcare Students at a Glance, Second Edition. Ian Peate.
© 2022 John Wiley & Sons Ltd. Published 2022 by John Wiley & Sons Ltd.
Companion website: www.wiley.com/go/peate/anatomyandphysiology

Circle of Willis

The circle of Willis (circulus arteriosus cerebri) is an anastomotic system of arteries (Figure 13.1) that sits at the base of the brain. It is a junction of several important arteries, helping blood flow from both the front and back sections of the brain.

The 'circle' was named after Thomas Willis by his student Richard Lower. Willis was the author of *Cerebri Anatome*, a book describing and depicting this vascular ring. Although such a vascular ring had been described earlier, the name Willis has been eponymously reproduced.

The circle of Willis encircles the stalk of the pituitary gland, providing important communications between the blood supply of the forebrain and hindbrain. The circle of Willis is formed when the internal carotid artery enters the cranial cavity bilaterally and then divides into the anterior cerebral and middle cerebral arteries. The anterior cerebral arteries are then united by an anterior communicating artery. These connections form the anterior half (anterior circulation) of the circle of Willis.

Posteriorly, the basilar artery, formed by the left and right vertebral arteries, branches into a left and right posterior cerebral artery, forming the posterior circulation. The posterior communicating arteries complete the circle of Willis by joining the internal carotid system anteriorly via the posterior communicating arteries.

Although in an adult the brain represents only 2% of total body weight, it uses 20% of oxygen and glucose even when at rest. When activities in a certain area of the brain increase, blood flow to that region will also increase. Even a momentary slowing of blood flow to the brain can result in unconsciousness.

Further decreases in blood flow, for a couple of minutes, can lead to impaired neuronal function. If the blood flow is restricted for 4 minutes or more, this may lead to permanent brain damage. As the brain does not store glucose, it is essential that there be a continuous supply of glucose to the brain.

Function of the circle of Willis

The circle of Willis provides numerous paths for the oxygenated blood to supply the brain. If any of the principal suppliers of oxygenated blood (i.e. the vertebral and internal carotid arteries) are constricted by physical pressure, occluded by disease or interrupted by injury, this could result in serious complications. The goal of treatment is to reduce the risk of stroke. Treatment options vary according to the severity of the arterial narrowing and whether the person is experiencing stroke-like symptoms or not.

The blood–brain barrier

The blood–brain barrier is a highly selective semi-permeable border; that is, it allows some materials to cross the barrier but will prevent others from crossing. In most parts of the body, the smallest blood vessels, called the capillaries, are lined with endothelial cells. Endothelial tissue has small spaces between each individual cell so that substances can move readily between the inside and outside of the vessel. However, in the brain, the endothelial cells fit tightly together (they are wedged together) and substances are not able to pass out of the bloodstream (Figure 13.2), providing an endothelial tight junction. Some molecules, for example glucose, are transported out of the blood by special methods.

Glial cells (astrocytes) form a layer around brain blood vessels and may be important in development of the blood–brain barrier. Astrocytes may also be responsible for transporting ions from the brain to the blood.

Function of the blood–brain barrier

The blood–brain barrier protects cells of the brain from harmful substances and pathogens by preventing passage of many substances from the blood into the brain tissue. It also provides a constant environment for the brain and protects it from hormones and neurotransmitters in the rest of the body.

The purpose of the blood–brain barrier is to protect against circulating toxins or pathogens that may cause brain infections, while at the same time allowing vital nutrients to reach the brain. It has a protective function.

A few water-soluble substances, such as glucose, cross the blood–brain barrier by active transport. Other substances, for example urea and most ions, cross the barrier very slowly. Protein and most antibiotics do not cross the barrier preventing them from entering brain tissue. However, lipid-soluble substances such as oxygen, carbon dioxide, alcohol and most anaesthetic drugs do cross the blood–brain barrier easily.

The blood–brain barrier can be broken down by hypertension (high blood pressure). Exposure to microwaves or radiation, infection and injury to the brain such as trauma, inflammation and ischaemia can all open the blood–brain barrier. The barrier is not considered to affect the movement of inflammatory cells into the CNS; activated lymphocytes can enter the normal CNS.

Clinical practice point

A cerebral aneurysm is a bulge or ballooning in a blood vessel in the brain. It looks like a berry hanging on a stem. A cerebral aneurysm can leak or rupture, which can cause bleeding into the brain (haemorrhagic stroke). Cerebral aneurysms generally rupture in the space between the brain and the thin tissues that cover the brain. This type of haemorrhagic stroke is known as a subarachnoid haemorrhage. A ruptured aneurysm will quickly become life-threatening and requires prompt medical treatment. A sudden, severe headache is the key symptom of a ruptured aneurysm, often described as the 'worst headache' ever experienced. Common signs and symptoms of a ruptured aneurysm include sudden, extremely severe headache, nausea and vomiting, neck stiffness, visual disturbance, photophobia, seizure, drooping eyelid (ptosis), loss of consciousness and confusion

14 The autonomic nervous system

Figure 14.1 The sympathetic and parasympathetic nervous systems.

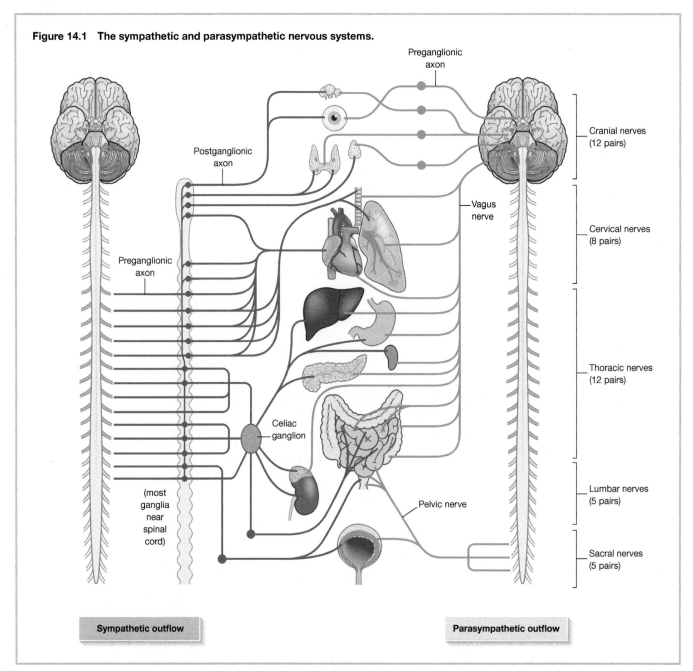

The autonomic nervous system (ANS) has a key role to play in the maintenance of homeostasis as it regulates the body's automatic, involuntary functions and, in common with the rest of the nervous system, consists of neurons, neuroglia and other connective tissue. Its structure, however, is unique in that it is divided into two parts: the sympathetic division and the parasympathetic division. Most autonomic responses cannot be consciously altered or suppressed to any great degree.

Sympathetic nervous system

The sympathetic division includes nerve fibres arising from the 12 thoracic and first two lumbar segments of the spinal cord; thus it is also referred to as the thoracolumbar division. The sympathetic division takes control of many internal organs when a stressful situation occurs. This can take the form of physical stress, for example if undertaking strenuous exercise, or emotional stress such as at times of anger or anxiety. In emergency situations, the sympathetic nervous system releases norepinephrine that assists in the 'fight or flight' response.

As with other parts of the nervous system, the sympathetic nervous system (SNS) operates through a series of interconnected neurons. Sympathetic neurons are often considered part of the peripheral nervous system, although there are many that lie within the central nervous system (CNS). Sympathetic neurons of the spinal cord (which is part of the CNS) communicate with peripheral sympathetic neurons through a series of sympathetic ganglia. Within the ganglia, spinal cord sympathetic neurons join peripheral sympathetic neurons through chemical synapses.

Spinal cord sympathetic neurons are called presynaptic (or preganglionic) neurons, while peripheral sympathetic neurons are known as postsynaptic (or postganglionic) neurons. At synapses within the sympathetic ganglia, preganglionic sympathetic neurons release acetylcholine, which is a chemical messenger binding and activating nicotinic acetylcholine receptors on postganglionic neurons.

Functions

The nerves of the sympathetic division speed up heart rate, dilate pupils, relax the bladder, increase blood pressure, increase respiration, dilate the blood vessels to the heart, increase blood flow to muscles, release epinephrine, release stored energy (glycogen), increase perspiration, decrease blood to the skin and slow down the GI tract.

Parasympathetic nervous system

The parasympathetic division includes fibres that arise from the lower end of the spinal cord and includes several cranial nerves; it is often referred to as the craniosacral division. The para sympathetic division is most active when the body is at rest it uses acetylcholine to control all the internal responses associated with a state of relaxation (Figure 14.1) and as such has many opposite effects on the body to the sympathetic nervous system.

In contrast to the 'flight or fight' activities of the sympathetic division, the parasympathetic division heightens 'rest and digest'. The parasympathetic responses support body functions that conserve and restore body energy during times of rest and recovery.

The parasympathetic nervous system (PNS) is composed of four cranial nerves originating from the brainstem. PNS activity begins in the head in the sacral region, which is why this activity is called craniosacral in nature, while the SNS is thoracolumbar in nature. The nerve most involved in PNS activity is the vagus nerve. This works by transmitting information between the posterior hypothalamus, the brainstem of the central nervous system and vital organs as well as the glands. The PNS works by antagonising the action of the SNS by lowering heart rate, decreasing blood pressure, constricting pupils and increasing intestinal motility. It increases the release of endorphin, a 'feel good' hormone, so we can recover from the actions caused by SNS stimulation.

Functions

Parasympathetic nervous system functions are as follows.

- Decreases heart rate and blood pressure
- Slows breathing
- Lubricates mouth and eyes
- Stimulates digestion and the storing of energy
- Constricts pupils
- Responsible for elimination

Autonomic control by the CNS

The hypothalamus is the major control and integration centre of the ANS. The hypothalamus receives sensory input related to visceral function, smell, taste, temperature and osmolality of blood. It also receives information about emotions from the limbic system. The output from the hypothalamus influences the autonomic centres in the brainstem (cardiac, respiration, salivation centres) as well as the spinal cord (defaecation, urination reflex centres).

Anatomically, the hypothalamus is connected to both the sympathetic and parasympathetic divisions. For example, stimulation of the sympathetic division increases the heart rate while the parasympathetic division will reduce the heart rate.

Autonomic reflexes

Autonomic reflexes occur when nerve impulses pass through an autonomic reflex arc. These have an important part to play in regulating controlled conditions in the body; for example, blood pressure regulation takes place by altering the heart rate, the force of ventricular contraction and vascular diameter.

The components for an autonomic reflex arc include a receptor (responding to a stimulus and producing a change that will ultimately trigger nerve impulses), sensory neuron (conducts nerve impulses from receptors to the CNS), integrating centre (located in the hypothalamus and spinal cord), motor neurons (impulses from the CNS pass along the motor neuron to the effector) and an effector (smooth muscle, cardiac muscle and glands).

Clinical practice point

Generalised anxiety disorder (GAD) is a mental health disorder producing fear, worry and a continual feeling of being overwhelmed. It is characterised by excessive, persistent and unrealistic worry about everyday things. Consider the following when making a diagnosis of GAD.
- The presence of excessive anxiety and worry that is difficult to control, easily moving from one topic to another.
- The anxiety and worry are accompanied by physical or cognitive symptoms, such as edginess or restlessness, tiring easily; more fatigued than usual, impaired concentration or feeling as though the mind goes blank, irritability, increased muscle aches or soreness, difficulty sleeping, a feeling of dread.

15 The peripheral nervous system

Figure 15.1 **The somatic nervous system.**

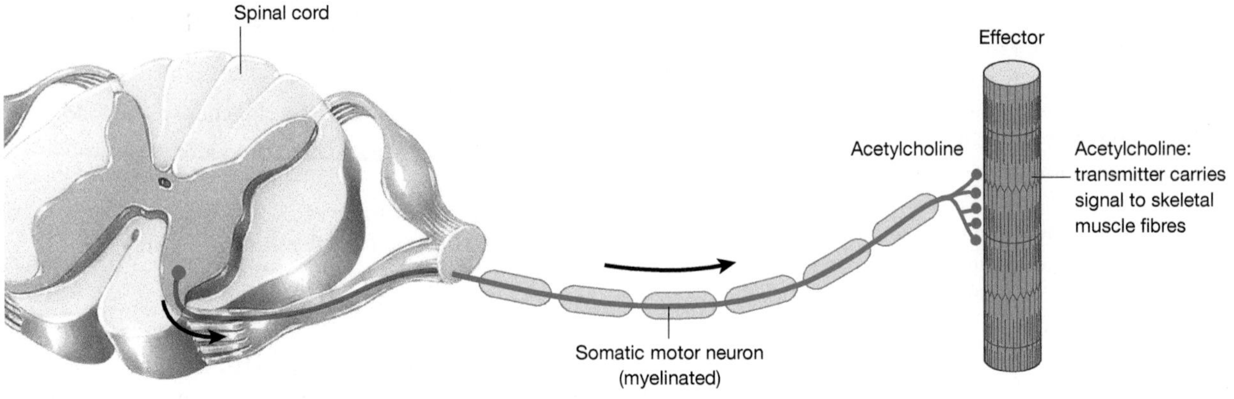
Spinal cord
Effector
Acetylcholine
Acetylcholine: transmitter carries signal to skeletal muscle fibres
Somatic motor neuron (myelinated)

Figure 15.2 **The motor pathway.**

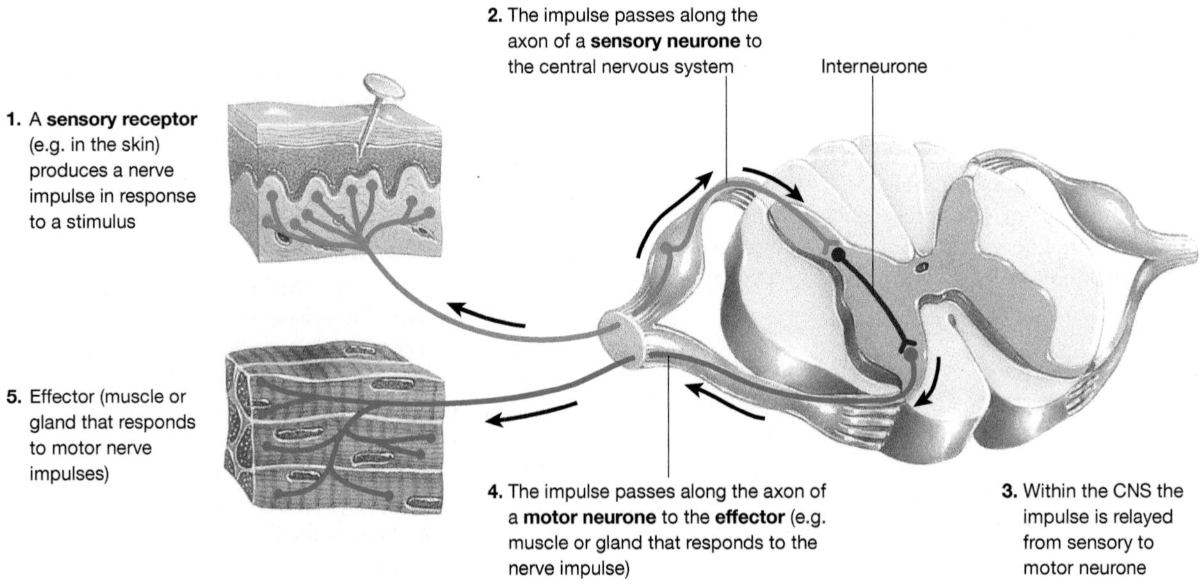
2. The impulse passes along the axon of a sensory neurone to the central nervous system
Interneurone
1. A sensory receptor (e.g. in the skin) produces a nerve impulse in response to a stimulus
5. Effector (muscle or gland that responds to motor nerve impulses)
4. The impulse passes along the axon of a motor neurone to the effector (e.g. muscle or gland that responds to the nerve impulse)
3. Within the CNS the impulse is relayed from sensory to motor neurone

Anatomy and Physiology for Nursing and Healthcare Students at a Glance, Second Edition. Ian Peate.

Companion website: www.wiley.com/go/peate/anatomyandphysiology

The peripheral nervous system (PNS) includes all the tissues that lie outside the central nervous system (CNS). These include cranial nerves, spinal cord, spinal nerves and autonomic system. There are two types of cells in the peripheral nervous system. These cells carry information to (sensory nervous cells) and from (motor nervous cells) the CNS. Cells of the sensory nervous system send information to the CNS from internal organs or from external stimuli.

Motor nervous system cells carry information from the CNS to organs, muscles and glands. The motor nervous system is divided into the somatic nervous system and the autonomic nervous system. The somatic nervous system has control over skeletal muscle and external sensory organs such as the skin. This system is said to be voluntary because the responses can be controlled consciously. Reflex reactions of skeletal muscle, however, are an exception. These are involuntary reactions to external stimuli.

Peripheral nervous system connections

The peripheral nervous system makes connections with various organs and structures of the body, established through cranial nerves and spinal nerves. There are 12 pairs of cranial nerves in the brain that create connections in the head and upper body, while 31 pairs of spinal nerves do the same for the rest of the body. While some cranial nerves contain only sensory neurons, most of the cranial nerves and all of the spinal nerves contain both motor and sensory neurons.

Sensory division

The sensory (afferent) division carries sensory signals by way of afferent nerve fibres from receptors in the CNS. It can be further subdivided into somatic and visceral divisions. The somatic sensory division transmits signals from receptors in the skin, muscles, bones and joints. The visceral sensory division transports signals mainly from the viscera of the thoracic and abdominal cavities.

Somatic

The somatic nervous system (Figure 15.1) is the part of the nervous system that has responsibility for voluntary body movement and sensing external stimuli. All five senses are controlled by the somatic nervous system. The somatic nervous system is a subpart of the peripheral nervous system.

The somatic nervous system consists of sensory neurons that conduct impulses from somatic and special sense receptors to the CNS and motor neurons from the CNS to skeletal muscles attached to the bone used for voluntary movement and sensory organs, including the eyes, ears, tongue and skin. In movement, the somatic nervous system carries impulses from the brain to the muscle to be moved, while in its sensory capacity, the somatic nervous system takes impulses from the sensory organ to the brain. There are therefore two portions, or limbs, of the somatic nervous system: the afferent and the efferent. The afferent, or sensory, neurons carry impulses from sense organs into the CNS, while the efferent, or motor, neurons carry impulses from the CNS to the muscles.

Visceral

The visceral division supplies and receives fibres to and from smooth muscle, cardiac muscle and glands. The visceral motor fibres (those that supply smooth muscle, cardiac muscle and glands) make up the autonomic nervous system (ANS). The ANS is composed of two divisions (see also Chapter 14).

- Parasympathetic division – this is important for the control of 'normal' body functions, for example, the normal operation of the digestive system.
- Sympathetic division – this is also called the 'fight or flight' division; it is important in helping us to cope with stress.

Motor division

The motor (efferent) division transports motor signals by way of efferent nerve fibres from the CNS to effectors (primarily glands and muscles) (Figure 15.2). It can be further divided into somatic and visceral divisions. The somatic motor division carrys signals to the skeletal muscles. The visceral motor division, which is also known as the autonomic nervous system, carries signals to glands, cardiac muscle and smooth muscle. It can be further subdivided into sympathetic and parasympathetic divisions.

Clinical practice point

Peripheral neuropathy occurs when nerves in the body's extremities, for example the hands, feet and arms, are damaged. Symptoms will depend on which nerves are affected. The main symptoms of peripheral neuropathy can include numbness and tingling in the feet or hands, a burning, stabbing or shooting pain in affected areas, loss of balance and co-ordination, and muscle weakness, particularly in the feet. These symptoms are normally constant, but they can come and go. If the underlying cause of peripheral neuropathy is not treated, the person may develop potentially serious complications, for example a foot ulcer that becomes infected. This could lead to gangrene if left untreated, which in severe cases could mean that the foot may have to be amputated. Peripheral neuropathy can also affect the nerves that control the automatic functions of the heart and circulation system, known as cardiovascular autonomic neuropathy.

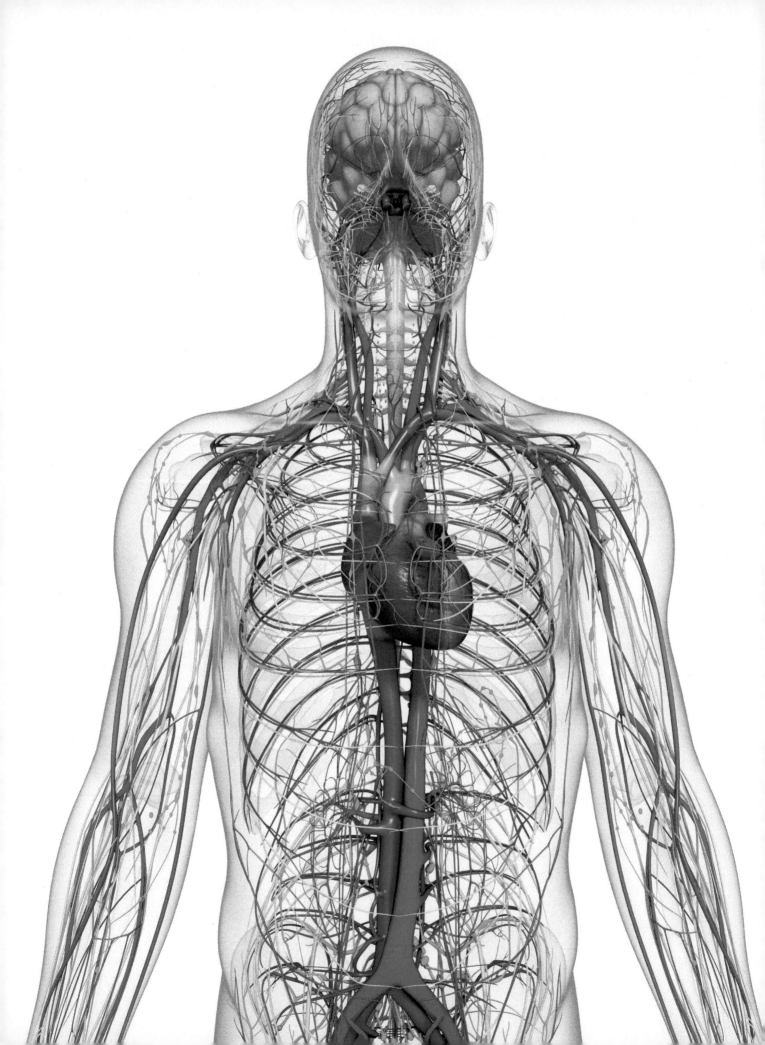

The heart and vascular system

Part 3

Chapters

16 The heart

Figure 16.1   The location of the heart.

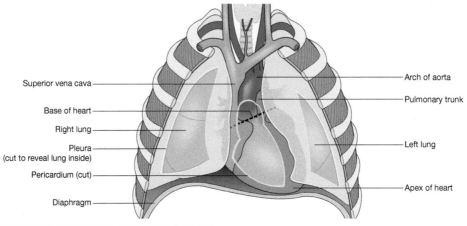

Superior vena cava

Base of heart

Right lung

Pleura
(cut to reveal lung inside)

Pericardium (cut)

Diaphragm

Arch of aorta

Pulmonary trunk

Left lung

Apex of heart

Source: Peate I, Wild K & Nair M (eds). Nursing Practice: Knowledge and Care (2014).

Figure 16.2   The walls of the heart.

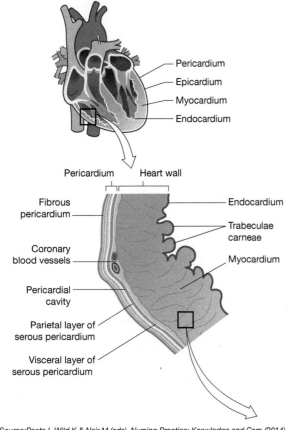

Pericardium

Epicardium

Myocardium

Endocardium

Pericardium   Heart wall

Fibrous
pericardium

Coronary
blood vessels

Pericardial
cavity

Parietal layer of
serous pericardium

Visceral layer of
serous pericardium

Endocardium

Trabeculae
carneae

Myocardium

Source:Peate I, Wild K & Nair M (eds). Nursing Practice: Knowledge and Care (2014).

Figure 16.3   Cells of the myocardium.

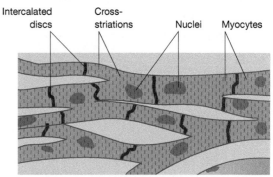

Intercalated
discs

Cross-
striations

Nuclei

Myocytes

Source: Peate I, Wild K & Nair M (eds). Nursing Practice: Knowledge and Care (2014).

Figure 16.4   Myocardial cells.

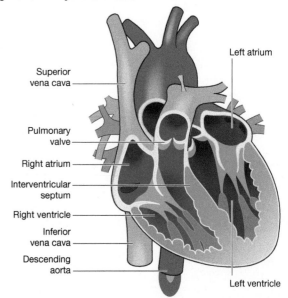

Superior
vena cava

Pulmonary
valve

Right atrium

Interventricular
septum

Right ventricle

Inferior
vena cava

Descending
aorta

Left atrium

Left ventricle

Source: Peate I, Wild K & Nair M (eds). Nursing Practice: Knowledge and Care (2014).

Anatomy and Physiology for Nursing and Healthcare Students at a Glance, Second Edition. Ian Peate.
© 2022 John Wiley & Sons Ltd. Published 2022 by John Wiley & Sons Ltd.
Companion website: www.wiley.com/go/peate/anatomyandphysiology

The heart is part of the cardiovascular system. It weighs approximately 250–390 g in men and 200–275 g in women and is a little larger than the owner's closed fist, being about 12 cm long and 9 cm wide. It is located in the thoracic cavity (chest) in the mediastinum (between the lungs), behind and to the left of the sternum (breastbone) (Figure 16.1). The heart rests on the diaphragm in the thoracic cavity.

Walls of the heart

Pericardium

A membrane called the pericardium (peri = around) surrounds the heart. This is referred to as a single sac surrounding the heart but is in fact made up of two sacs (fibrous pericardium and serous pericardium) that are closely connected to each other (Figure 16.2). These two sacs have very different structures.

Fibrous pericardium

This is a tough, inelastic layer made up of dense, irregular, connective tissue. Its purpose is to prevent overstretching of the heart. It also provides protection to the heart and anchors it in place.

Serous pericardium

The serous pericardium is a thinner, more delicate structure which forms a double layer around the heart. The outer layer is fused to the fibrous pericardium. The visceral pericardium (otherwise known as the epicardium) adheres tightly to the surface of the heart.

Myocardium

The myocardium makes up the majority of the bulk of the heart. It is a muscle that is only found within the heart, specialised in its structure and function. The work of the myocardium can be divided into two parts: the majority of the myocardium is specialised to undertake mechanical work (contraction); the remainder is specialised to undertake the task of initiating and conducting electrical impulses. The cardiac muscle cells (myocytes) are held together in interlacing bundles of fibres arranged in a spiral or in circular bundles (Figure 16.3).

Myocardial thickness varies between the four chambers of the heart. The ventricles have thicker walls than the atria; however, the left ventricle has the thickest myocardial wall. This is because the left ventricle has to pump blood great distances to parts of the body at a higher pressure and the resistance to blood flow is greater.

Endocardium

This is the innermost layer that is made up of endothelium overlying a thin layer of connective tissue. The endothelium is continuous with the endothelial lining of the large vessels of the heart. It also provides a lining to allow the blood to flow through the chambers smoothly.

Chambers of the heart

There are four chambers in the heart: two atria (left and right; the singular of atria is atrium) and two ventricles (left and right). On the anterior surface of each of the atria is a wrinkled pouch-like structure called an auricle. The main function of the auricle is to increase the volume of blood in the atrium. Between the ventricles is a dividing wall, the intraventricular septum (Figure 16.4). Thus

with the septum between the atria and the septum between the ventricles, there is no mixing of blood between the two sides.

Valves of the heart

Between the atria and the ventricles there are two valves (the atrioventricular valves).

- The tricuspid valve – this is made up of three cusps (leaflets) and it lies between the right atrium and the right ventricle.
- The bicuspid (mitral) valve – this is made up of two cusps and it lies between the left atrium and the left ventricle.

The purpose of the atrioventricular valves is to prevent the backward flow of blood from the ventricles into the atria.

Blood vessels of the heart

The aorta is the largest blood vessel of the heart; it is also the largest blood vessel in the body. It is the aorta that carries and distributes oxygen-rich blood to all arteries. The coronary arteries are the first blood vessels that branch off from the ascending aorta. The coronary arteries supply richly oxygenated and nutrient-filled blood to the heart muscle (the myocardium). There are two main coronary arteries: right coronary artery and left coronary artery. Other arteries diverge from these two main arteries and they extend to the lower portion of the heart.

The pulmonary arteries are unique in that, unlike most arteries which transport oxygenated blood to other parts of the body, the pulmonary arteries transport deoxygenated blood to the lungs. After picking up oxygen in the lungs, the oxygen-rich blood is then returned to the heart via the pulmonary veins.

There are four pulmonary veins which extend from the left atrium to the lungs. They are the:

- right superior vein
- right inferior vein
- left superior vein
- left inferior pulmonary vein.

The venae cavae (superior and inferior) (singular vena cava) are the two largest veins in the body. These blood vessels carry deoxygenated blood from the various regions of the body to the right atrium of the heart. As the deoxygenated blood is returned to the heart and continues to flow through the cardiac cycle, it is transported to the lungs where it will become oxygenated. The blood then travels back to the heart and from here it is pumped out to the rest of the body via the aorta. The oxygen-depleted blood is returned to the heart again via the venae cavae.

Clinical practice point

A myocardial infarction is a sudden blockage of blood flow to the heart. Without adequate blood flow, the heart muscle will not receive the nutrients and oxygen that it needs in order to function effectively. Symptoms include chest pain or discomfort, a heaviness, tightness, pressure, aching, burning, numbness, fullness or squeezing feeling lasting for more than a few minutes or which goes away and returns, pain or discomfort in other areas of the upper body including the arms, left shoulder, back, neck, jaw or stomach, breathing difficulties, heartburn, nausea, sweating. Most women and men report symptoms of chest pain with a myocardial infarction; women may report unusual symptoms, such as upper back or shoulder pain, jaw pain or pain spreading to the jaw, pressure or pain in the center of the chest, light-headedness, pain radiating to the arm, unusual fatigue for several days. Call emergency services immediately – the earlier the treatment, the better the outcome.

17 Blood flow through the heart

Figure 17.1   Blood flow through the heart.

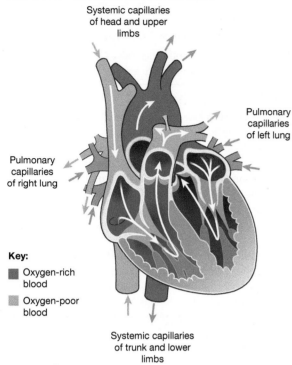

Systemic capillaries
of head and upper
limbs

Pulmonary
capillaries
of left lung

Pulmonary
capillaries
of right lung

Key:

■ Oxygen-rich
blood

■ Oxygen-poor
blood

Systemic capillaries
of trunk and lower
limbs

Source: Peate I, Wild K & Nair M (eds). Nursing Practice: Knowledge and Care (2014).

Figure 17.2   The blood vessels of the heart.

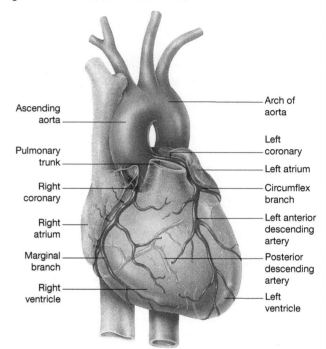

Ascending
aorta

Pulmonary
trunk

Right
coronary

Right
atrium

Marginal
branch

Right
ventricle

Arch of
aorta

Left
coronary

Left atrium

Circumflex
branch

Left anterior
descending
artery

Posterior
descending
artery

Left
ventricle

Source: Peate I, Wild K & Nair M (eds). Nursing Practice: Knowledge and Care (2014).

Figure 17.3   The coronary veins.

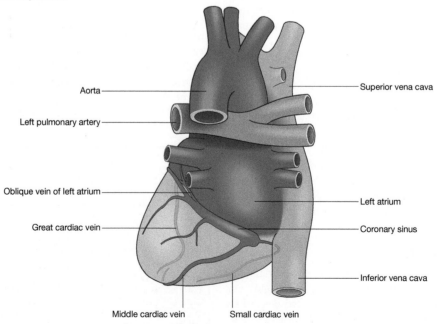

Aorta

Left pulmonary artery

Oblique vein of left atrium

Great cardiac vein

Superior vena cava

Left atrium

Coronary sinus

Inferior vena cava

Middle cardiac vein   Small cardiac vein

Anatomy and Physiology for Nursing and Healthcare Students at a Glance, Second Edition. Ian Peate.
© 2022 John Wiley & Sons Ltd. Published 2022 by John Wiley & Sons Ltd.
Companion website: www.wiley.com/go/peate/anatomyandphysiology

Blood flow

The body's circulatory system has three distinct parts: pulmonary circulation, coronary circulation and systemic circulation – in other words, the lungs (pulmonary), the heart (coronary) and the rest of the system (systemic). Each distinct part must be working independently in order for them to all work together in an effective way.

Pulmonary circulation

The pulmonary circulation is a system of blood vessels that forms a closed circuit between the heart and the lungs.

The blood enters the heart through two large veins, the inferior and superior vena cava, emptying oxygen-poor blood from the body into the right atrium. Blood flows from the right atrium into the right ventricle through the open tricuspid valve. When the ventricles are full, the tricuspid valve will shut. This will prevent the blood from flowing backwards into the atria while the ventricles contract (squeeze).

Once the blood travels through the pulmonary valve, it then enters the lungs. This is called the pulmonary circulation. From the pulmonary valve, blood travels to the pulmonary artery to the tiny capillary vessels in the lungs. Here, oxygen travels from the tiny air sacs in the lungs, through the walls of the capillaries, into the blood. At the same time, carbon dioxide, a waste product of metabolism, will pass from the blood into the air sacs. Carbon dioxide then leaves the body as we exhale. Once the blood is oxygenated, it will then travel back to the left atrium through the pulmonary veins (Figure 17.1).

Systemic circulation

The systemic circulation is the circuit of vessels that supplies oxygenated blood to and returns deoxygenated blood from the tissues of the body. The pulmonary vein empties oxygen-rich blood from the lungs into the left atrium.

Blood leaves the heart through the aortic valve, into the aorta and then to the body (the systemic circulation). This pattern is repeated, causing the blood to flow continuously to the heart, lungs and body (see Figure 17.1).

The powerful contraction of the heart's left ventricle forces the blood into the aorta which then branches into many smaller arteries which run throughout the body. The inside layer of an artery is very smooth, which allows the blood to flow quickly. The outside layer of an artery is very strong, enabling the blood to flow forcefully. The oxygen-rich blood enters the capillaries where the oxygen and nutrients are then released. The waste products are collected and the waste-rich blood flows into the veins so as to circulate back to the heart where pulmonary circulation will allow the exchange of gases in the lungs to occur.

Coronary circulation

The heart itself receives about 5% of the body's blood supply. It is essential that the heart receives a plentiful supply of blood to ensure the constant supply of oxygen and nutrients and the efficient removal of waste products required by the myocardium so that it can perform at an optimum level.

Nutrients from the blood cannot diffuse quickly from the chambers of the heart to supply the cells of the heart. Only the inner part of the endocardium (this is about 2 mm in thickness) is supplied with blood directly from the inside of the heart chambers. The rest of the heart's blood supply is supplied by the coronary arteries. The coronary arteries come directly off the aorta, just after the aortic valve. They continuously divide into smaller branches and form a web of blood vessels to supply the heart muscle (Figure 17.2).

Coronary arteries

The entire body must be supplied with nutrients and oxygen via the circulatory system and the heart is no exception. The coronary circulation refers to the vessels that supply and drain the heart. Coronary arteries are so named due to the way they encircle the heart, much like a crown.

The coronary arteries supply blood to the heart muscle (myocardium). As with all other tissues in the body, the heart muscle requires oxygen-rich blood in order for it to function, and oxygen-depleted blood has to be carried away.

The coronary arteries branch from the ascending aorta and encircle the heart like a crown. As the coronary arteries are compressed during each heart beat, the blood does not flow through the coronary arteries at this time. Thus blood flow to the myocardium occurs during the relaxation phase of the cardiac cycle, which is the opposite to every other part of the body.

The left coronary artery divides into the anterior interventricular, branch, which supplies oxygenated blood to both ventricles, and the circumflex branch, which distributes oxygenated blood to the left ventricle and left atrium. The right coronary artery, which divides into the right posterior descending and acute marginal arteries, supplies oxygenated blood to the right atrium and both the ventricles, sinoatrial node (cluster of cells in the right atrial wall that regulates the heart's rhythmic rate) and atrioventricular node.

Coronary veins

The coronary veins return deoxygenated blood (containing metabolic waste products) from the myocardium to the right atrium. This blood then flows back to the lungs for reoxygenation and removal of carbon dioxide.

Coronary veins contain valves that prevent back flow; a Thebesian valve may or may not cover the ostium (opening) of the coronary sinus. Typically cardiac veins are free of atherosclerotic plaques. The coronary sinus is a collection of veins joined together to form a large vessel that collects blood from the heart muscle (myocardium) (Figure 17.3). It delivers deoxygenated blood to the right atrium.

The coronary sinus opens into the right atrium, at the coronary sinus orifice, between the inferior vena cava and the right atrioventricular orifice. It returns the blood from the substance of the heart, and is protected by a semi-circular fold of the lining membrane of the auricle.

Clinical practice point

Coronary heart disease (CHD) is a major cause of death in the UK and globally. CHD is sometimes also called ischaemic heart disease or coronary artery disease. CHD is the term that describes what happens when the heart's blood supply is blocked or interrupted by a build-up of fatty substances in the coronary arteries. Over time, the walls of the arteries can become furred up with fatty deposits. This process is called atherosclerosis and the fatty deposits are known as atheroma. Atherosclerosis can be caused by lifestyle factors, that include smoking and regularly drinking excessive amounts of alcohol. The main symptoms of CHD include angina (chest pain), shortness of breath (dyspnoea), pain throughout the body, feeling faint (syncope) and nausea. Not everybody will have the same symptoms of CHD and some people may not have any symptoms before coronary heart disease is diagnosed.

18 The conducting system

Figure 18.1   The conducting system of the heart.

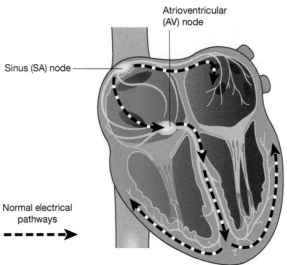

Atrioventricular
(AV) node

Sinus (SA) node

Normal electrical
pathways

Source: Peate I, Wild K & Nair M (eds). Nursing Practice: Knowledge and Care (2014).

Figure 18.2   The cardiac cycle.

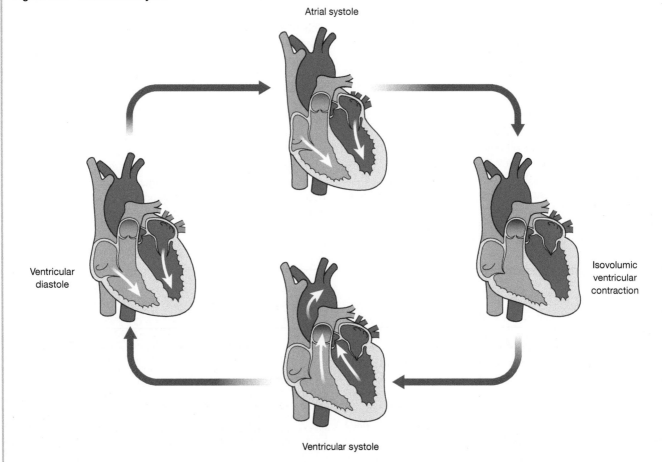

Atrial systole

Ventricular
diastole

Isovolumic
ventricular
contraction

Ventricular systole

Cardiac conduction

The cardiac conduction system is composed of a collection of nodes and specialised conduction cells that initiate and co-ordinate contraction of the heart muscle.

Cardiac conduction is the rate at which the heart conducts electrical impulses. These impulses usually result in the heart contracting and then relaxing. The constant cycle of heart muscle contraction followed by relaxation causes the blood to be pumped throughout the body. The conduction pathway is made up of five elements:

- sinoatrial node
- atrioventricular node
- bundle of His
- left and right bundle branches
- Purkinje fibres.

Sinoatrial node

The sinoatrial (SA) node is the natural pacemaker of the heart, located in the right atrium (see Figure 18.1). The SA node is a spindle-shaped structure composed of a fibrous tissue matrix with closely packed specialist cells. The SA node releases electrical stimuli at a regular rate. The rate at which they are released is determined by the needs of the body. Each stimulus passes through the myocardial cells of the atria, creating a wave of contraction which spreads at speed through both atria.

The heart is composed of around half a billion cells. The majority of the cells make up the ventricular walls. The rapidity of atrial contraction is such that around 100 million myocardial cells contract in less than one-third of a second, so fast that the contraction of the atria appears instantaneous.

Atrioventricular node

The atrioventricular (AV) node is situated on the right side of the partition that divides the atria, close to the bottom of the right atrium (see Figure 18.1). When impulses from the SA node reach the AV node, they are delayed for about a tenth of a second. This delay permits the atria to contract and empty their contents first. The AV node regulates the signals to the ventricles, preventing rapid conduction (atrial fibrillation), as well as making sure that the atria are empty and closed before stimulating the ventricles.

Bundle of His

The bundle of His (also known as the atrioventricular bundle) is a collection of heart muscle cells specialised for electrical conduction that transmits the electrical impulses from the AV node to the point of the apex of the fascicular branches. This bundle is the only site where action potentials can conduct from the atria to the ventricles.

Left and right bundle branches

These are the parts of the network of specialised conducting fibres that transmit electrical impulses within the ventricles of the heart. Bundle branches are a continuation of the AV bundle, which extends from the upper part of the intraventricular septum. The AV bundle divides into a left and a right branch, each going to its respective ventricle by passing down the septum and below the endocardium. Within the ventricles, the bundle branches subdivide and terminate in the Purkinje fibres.

Purkinje fibres

This network of specialised cells is rich with glycogen and has extensive gap junctions. These fibres are located in the inner ventricular walls of the heart. They consist of specialised cardiomyocytes that are able to conduct cardiac action potentials more quickly and efficiently than any other cells in the heart. Purkinje fibres allow the heart's conduction system to create synchronised contractions of its ventricles, and are therefore essential for maintaining a consistent heart rhythm.

The cardiac cycle

The cardiac cycle is the sequence of events that occurs when the heart beats (Figure 18.2). There are two phases of the cardiac cycle. In the diastole phase, the ventricles are relaxed and the heart fills with blood. In the systole phase, the ventricles contract and pump blood to the arteries. One cardiac cycle is completed when the heart fills with blood and the blood is pumped out of the heart.

First diastole phase

During the diastole phase, the atria and ventricles are relaxed and the atrioventricular valves are open. Deoxygenated blood from the superior and inferior venae cavae flows into the right atrium. The open atrioventricular valves then permit the blood to pass through to the ventricles. The SA node contracts, which triggers the atria to contract. The right atrium empties its contents into the right ventricle. The tricuspid valve prevents the blood from flowing back into the right atrium.

First systole phase

During the first systole phase, the right ventricle receives impulses from the Purkinje fibres and it contracts. The atrioventricular valves close and the semilunar valves open. The deoxygenated blood is pumped into the pulmonary artery. The pulmonary valve prevents the blood from flowing back into the right ventricle. The pulmonary artery carries the blood to the lungs where gas exchange occurs. The oxygenated blood returns to the left atrium via the pulmonary veins.

Second diastole phase

In the next diastole period, the semilunar valves close and the atrioventricular valves open. Blood from the pulmonary veins fills the left atrium (blood from the venae cavae is also filling the right atrium.) The SA node contracts again which triggers the atria to contract. The left atrium empties its contents into the left ventricle. The mitral valve prevents the oxygenated blood from flowing back into the left atrium.

Second systole phase

During the following systole phase, the atrioventricular valves close and the semilunar valves open. The left ventricle receives impulses from the Purkinje fibres and contracts. Oxygenated blood is pumped into the aorta. The aortic valve prevents the oxygenated blood from flowing back into the left ventricle. The aorta branches out, providing oxygenated blood to all parts of the body. The oxygen-depleted blood is returned to the heart via the venae cavae.

Clinical practice point

A cardiac pacemaker is an electronic device that provides electrical stimuli to the heart muscle. The function of the pacemaker (or pacer) is to maintain the heart rate when the patient's own intrinsic system cannot or does not do so. The electrical stimulus depolarises the heart and causes a contraction to occur at a controlled rate. The stimulus of the pacer is produced by a pulse generator and is delivered via electrodes or leads implanted in the epicardium or endocardium. The electrodes may be unipolar or bipolar and the proximal end attaches to a pulse generator that is placed in the chest or abdomen. Caring for people with pacemakers involves the monitoring and prevention of common complications, preventing dislodgement and offering education and advice to the person on the correct use and maintenance of the pacemaker.

19 Nerve supply to the heart

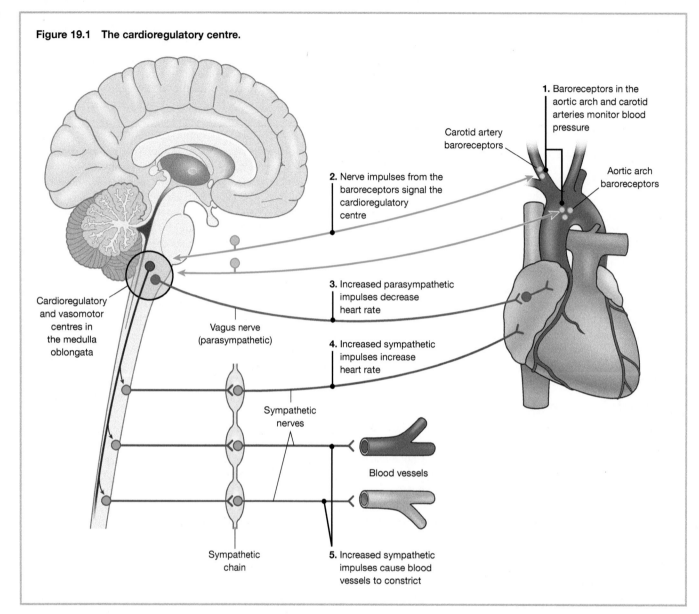

Figure 19.1   The cardioregulatory centre.

1. Baroreceptors in the aortic arch and carotid arteries monitor blood pressure

Carotid artery baroreceptors

Aortic arch baroreceptors

2. Nerve impulses from the baroreceptors signal the cardioregulatory centre

3. Increased parasympathetic impulses decrease heart rate

4. Increased sympathetic impulses increase heart rate

Cardioregulatory and vasomotor centres in the medulla oblongata

Vagus nerve (parasympathetic)

Sympathetic nerves

Sympathetic chain

Blood vessels

5. Increased sympathetic impulses cause blood vessels to constrict

Anatomy and Physiology for Nursing and Healthcare Students at a Glance, Second Edition. Ian Peate.
© 2022 John Wiley & Sons Ltd. Published 2022 by John Wiley & Sons Ltd.
Companion website: www.wiley.com/go/peate/anatomyandphysiology

The autonomic nervous system

Nervous system regulation of the heart originates in the cardioregulatory centre in the medulla oblongata (Figure 19.1). This region of the brainstem receives input from a variety of sensory receptors and from higher brain centres such as the limbic system and cerebral cortex.

When activated by a stimulus, such as exercise or stress, the sympathetic nerve fibres release norepinephrine at their cardiac endings as a neurotransmitter. This leads to the excitation of the sinoatrial node and an increase in its production of action potentials and thus an increase in heart rate.

Alternatively, when the parasympathetic nervous system is stimulated, this results in the release of acetylcholine at the parasympathetic cardiac nerve endings, which has the effect of reducing the rate of action potential generation in the sinoatrial node and thus reducing heart rate.

Both the sympathetic and parasympathetic nervous systems are active at all times but the parasympathetic nervous system normally has the dominant influence. This can be seen if the vagus nerve (cranial nerve X) is cut, for instance in heart transplant patients. In these situations the sinoatrial node will normally produce action potentials at a rate of 100 a minute and therefore the heart rate increases to 100 beats per minute. The removal of the influence of the parasympathetic nervous system (by disconnection of the vagus nerves) removes the heart rate-reducing effect of this system. The right vagus nerve primarily innervates the SA node, whereas the left vagus innervates the AV node; however, significant overlap can exist in the anatomical distribution.

Chemical regulation

There are certain chemicals that can influence the heart rate. Hypoxia, acidosis and alkalosis can all cause depression of cardiac activity.

Hormones

Epinephrine and norepinephrine from the adrenal glands increase heart rate and contractility. Stress, physical activity and excitement stimulate the adrenal glands to secrete more hormones, increasing the activity of the heart. Thyroid hormones from the thyroid gland also increase heart rate and contractility. These hormones affect cardiac muscle fibres in much the same way as norepinephrine by the sympathetic nervous system; they increase both heart rate and contractility.

Ions

The difference in the levels of cations between the intracellular and extracellular fluid is important for the production of action potentials in all nerve and muscle fibres, including the heart. For example, concentrations of potassium, sodium and calcium have a large effect on how the heart functions. An elevated level of potassium or sodium can decrease heart rate and contractility and cause cardiac dysfunction. An increase in intracellular calcium levels raises heart rate and also strengthens the heart beat. On the other hand, excess sodium blocks calcium entry into the cells and this can decrease the force of contraction, while excess potassium will block action potentials.

Baroreceptors

Baroreceptors are specialised mechanical receptors located in the carotid sinus and also the aortic arch; they are sensory cells. They are sensitive to the amount of stretch in these blood vessels and have direct outflow via the autonomic nervous system to the cardiovascular centre in the medulla oblongata.

The cardiovascular centre of the medulla oblongata is the main centre that controls autonomic nervous activity that affects the heart. The cardiovascular centre is made up of two subcentres.

Cardioinhibitory centre

This centre directly controls parasympathetic outflow to the heart (particularly the sinoatrial node), so increased outflow from this centre has the potential to reduce heart rate. The neurotransmitter acetylcholine directly stimulates the heart to decrease cardiac output, to return the circulatory system to a resting homeostasis after episodes of increased muscular activity or fight-or-flight emergencies. The cardioinhibitory centre plays the more minor role in controlling cardiac output.

Vasomotor centre

The vasomotor centre is divided into the pressor area and the depressor area. The pressor area has a relatively constant outflow of action potentials to the heart via the sympathetic nervous system. This has a direct effect on both heart rate and the force of ventricular contraction (and because of this, stroke volume) as well as effects on the vasculature which subsequently will affect heart function by changing preload and afterload. Outflow from the pressor area is moderated by nerves that transmit impulses from the depressor area which have a directly inhibiting effect on the transmission of impulses from the pressor area. Thus, it can be thought of that the nerve impulses of the depressor area act like a 'collar' or tap; the greater the number of impulses from the depressor area, the tighter the collar or tap is made, reducing the number of impulses from the pressor area to the heart and thus the effect on heart rate and force of contraction.

Other factors in heart regulation

Other factors that can affect heart rate include exercise, gender, body temperature and age.

Body temperature

Body temperature affects several processes in the body. When body temperature goes up, blood vessels dilate and this increases heart rate, in order to compensate for a drop in blood pressure. On the other hand, a decrease in temperature can lower the heart rate but only to some degree. If the temperature gets too low, the body will actually increase the heart rate, while trying to warm up.

Body fluid level

Dehydration decreases the amount of fluids in the blood which causes constriction of the coronary arteries. At the same time, the heart begins to beat faster, in order to push the thicker blood through the blood vessels.

Clinical practice point

Normal blood levels of potassium are critical for maintaining normal heart electrical rhythm. Both low blood potassium levels (hypokalaemia) and high blood potassium levels (hyperkalaemia) can lead to abnormal heart rhythms. The most important clinical effect of hyperkalaemia is related to electrical rhythm of the heart.

20 The structure of the blood vessels

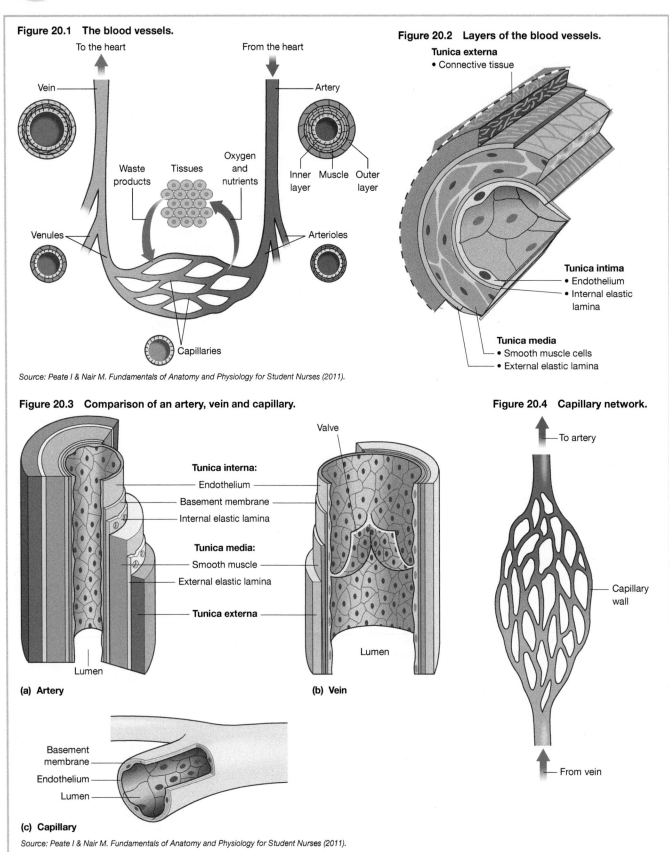

Figure 20.1   The blood vessels.

To the heart

From the heart

Vein

Artery

Waste products

Tissues

Oxygen and nutrients

Inner layer   Muscle   Outer layer

Venules

Arterioles

Capillaries

Source: Peate I & Nair M. Fundamentals of Anatomy and Physiology for Student Nurses (2011).

Figure 20.2   Layers of the blood vessels.

Tunica externa
• Connective tissue

Tunica intima
• Endothelium
• Internal elastic lamina

Tunica media
• Smooth muscle cells
• External elastic lamina

Figure 20.3   Comparison of an artery, vein and capillary.

Valve

Tunica interna:
Endothelium
Basement membrane
Internal elastic lamina

Tunica media:
Smooth muscle
External elastic lamina

Tunica externa

Lumen

Lumen

(a) Artery

(b) Vein

Basement membrane
Endothelium
Lumen

(c) Capillary

Source: Peate I & Nair M. Fundamentals of Anatomy and Physiology for Student Nurses (2011).

Figure 20.4   Capillary network.

To artery

Capillary wall

From vein

The average person has approximately 6 L of blood in their body. This blood is carried by several different types of blood vessels, each of which is specialised so as to play its role in circulating the blood around the body.

The blood vessels

Blood vessels are part of the circulatory system that transports blood throughout the body. There are three major types of blood vessels (Figure 20.1).

1 The arteries, carrying the blood away from the heart.
2 The capillaries, which enable the exchange of water, nutrients and chemicals between the blood and the tissues.
3 The veins, which carry blood from the capillaries back towards the heart.

All arteries, with the exception of the pulmonary and umbilical arteries, carry oxygenated blood, while most veins carry deoxygenated blood from the tissues back to the heart, with the exceptions of the pulmonary and umbilical veins, both of which carry oxygenated blood. The capillaries form the microcirculatory system and it is at this point that nutrients, gases, water and electrolytes are exchanged between the blood and the tissue fluid. Capillaries are tiny, extremely thin-walled vessels that act as a bridge between arteries and veins. The thin walls of the capillaries enable oxygen and nutrients to be passed from the blood into tissue fluid and allow waste products to pass from tissue fluid into the blood.

Structure of the blood vessels

Generally, the arterial system transports oxygenated blood from the heart and delivers it to the capillaries. In the capillaries, oxygen and nutrient exchange can occur.

The walls of the larger blood vessels consist of three layers (Figure 20.2).

1 The tunica intima consists of a thin layer of endothelial cells.
2 The tunica media contains smooth muscles and elastic fibres.
3 The tunica externa is an outer layer consisting of fibroblasts, nerves and collagenous tissue.

The endothelium is an epithelial lining that is only one cell thick. Therefore, the tunica interna is always very, very thin.

The arteries

Arteries receive blood under high pressure from the ventricles of the heart. They must therefore be able to stretch each time the heart beats, without collapsing under the increased pressure. The walls of arteries consist of three layers.

1 An outer layer.
2 A thick middle layer.
3 An inner layer.

The outer layer consists of white fibrous connective tissue which merges to the outside with the loose connective tissue. This helps to anchor the arteries because the heart pumps the blood through the arteries at great pressure. The thick middle layer consists of elastic connective tissue and involuntary muscle tissue. This layer is supplied with two sets of nerves: one that stimulates the muscles to relax so that the artery is permitted to widen, and the other stimulating the circular muscles to contract, which causes the artery to become narrower. The inner layer of endothelium is made up of flat epithelial cells packed closely together and continuous with the endocardium of the heart. The flat cells make the inside of the arteries smooth in order to limit friction between the blood flowing within the artery and the lining of the vessel.

The veins

The veins are the major vessels of the venous system. As veins carry blood back to the heart, the pressure exerted by the heart beat on them is much less than it is in the arteries. The middle muscular wall of a vein is therefore much thinner than that of an artery and generally the diameter is larger. Veins differ from arteries also in that they have semilunar valves which help to prevent the blood from flowing backwards (Figure 20.3).

The vein valves are necessary to keep blood flowing toward the heart, but they are also required to allow blood to flow against the force of gravity. For example, blood returning to the heart from the foot has to be able to flow up the leg. Generally, the force of gravity would discourage that from happening. The vein valves, however, provide 'footholds' for the blood as it flows its way up. The valves are like gates that only allow traffic to move in one direction. They also act together with muscle contraction, squeezing the veins and propelling blood towards the heart.

Veins receive blood from the capillaries after the exchange of oxygen and carbon dioxide has taken place. Therefore, the veins transport carbon dioxide-rich blood back to the lungs and heart. It is important that the carbon dioxide-rich blood keeps moving in the proper direction and is not allowed to flow backward; this is accomplished by the semilunar valves present in the veins.

The capillaries

Capillaries are tiny blood vessels, of approximately 5–20 micrometres diameter. There are networks of capillaries (Figure 20.4) in most of the organs and tissues of the body. The walls of capillaries are composed of only a single layer of cells, the endothelium. This layer is so thin that molecules such as oxygen, water and lipids can pass through it by diffusion and enter the tissues. Waste products such as carbon dioxide and urea can diffuse back into the blood to be carried away for removal from the body. Capillaries are so small that the red blood cells need to change their shape in order to pass through them in single file.

The flow of blood in the capillaries is controlled by structures known as precapillary sphincters. These are located between arterioles and capillaries, and contain muscle fibres that allow them to contract. When the sphincters are open, blood flows freely to the capillary beds of body tissue. When the sphincters are closed, blood cannot flow through the capillary beds. Fluid exchange between the capillaries and the body tissues takes place at the capillary bed.

Clinical practice point

A venous thromboembolism (VTE) refers to a blood clot forming in a vein which can partially or completely obstruct the flow of blood. VTE includes both deep vein thrombosis (DVT) and pulmonary embolism (PE). Hospital-acquired venous thromboembolism refers to a VTE that occurs within 90 days of hospital admission. It is a common and potentially preventable problem. The risk factors for VTE include surgery, trauma, significant immobility, malignancy, obesity, acquired or inherited hypercoagulable states, pregnancy and the postpartum period, and hormonal therapy (combined hormonal contraception or hormone replacement therapy).

A DVT, the most common form of VTE, usually occurs in the deep veins of the legs or pelvis but may affect other sites, for example the upper limbs and the intracranial and splanchnic veins. Symptoms of a DVT include unilateral localised pain, swelling, tenderness, skin changes and/or vein distension.

21 The blood pressure

Figure 21.1 The baroreceptors.

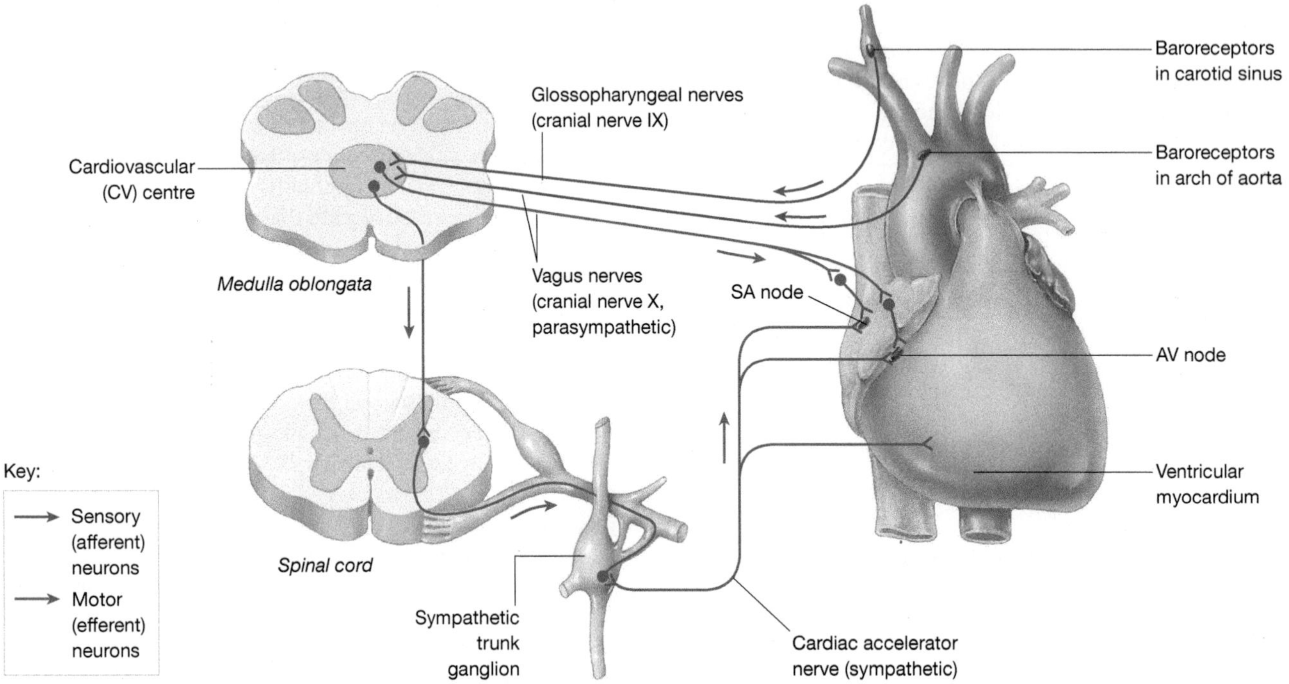

Cardiovascular (CV) centre

Medulla oblongata

Glossopharyngeal nerves (cranial nerve IX)

Vagus nerves (cranial nerve X, parasympathetic)

Baroreceptors in carotid sinus

Baroreceptors in arch of aorta

SA node

AV node

Ventricular myocardium

Key:

→ Sensory (afferent) neurons

→ Motor (efferent) neurons

Spinal cord

Sympathetic trunk ganglion

Cardiac accelerator nerve (sympathetic)

Source: Tortora GJ & Derrickson BH. Priniciples of Anatomy and Physiology 12e (2009).

Figure 21.2 Blood pressure measurement.

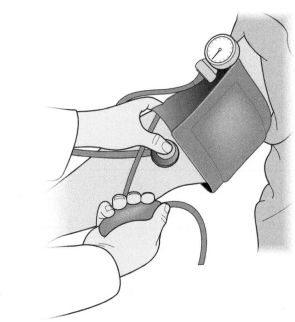

Anatomy and Physiology for Nursing and Healthcare Students at a Glance, Second Edition. Ian Peate.
© 2022 John Wiley & Sons Ltd. Published 2022 by John Wiley & Sons Ltd.
Companion website: www.wiley.com/go/peate/anatomyandphysiology

What is blood pressure?

Blood pressure is a measure of how well the cardiovascular system is functioning. Blood pressure has to be high enough to supply organs with blood and nutrients but not so high that blood vessels could become damaged. Therefore, the body has to maintain control over its blood pressure to keep it at a normal level. Blood pressure is the pressure exerted by blood within the blood vessel. The pressure is at its greatest nearer the heart but decreases as the blood moves away from the heart.

Three factors regulate blood pressure.

1. Neuronal regulation – through the autonomic nervous system.
2. Hormonal regulation – adrenaline, noradrenaline, renin and others.
3. Autoregulation – through the renin-angiotensin system.

Physiological factors

A number of physiological factors influence arterial blood pressure, which may also be affected by other factors such as age, gender, hormones, disease and exercise. The volume of blood that is present in the body affects blood pressure. An increase in blood volume increases the rate of blood flow to the heart, resulting in increased cardiac output.

Peripheral resistance is another physiological factor. In the circulatory system, this is the resistance of the blood vessels. The higher the resistance, the higher the arterial pressure upstream from the resistance to blood flow. Resistance is related to vessel radius (the larger the radius, the lower the resistance), vessel length (the longer the vessel, the higher the resistance), blood viscosity and the smoothness of the blood vessel walls. An increase in viscosity of the blood increases blood pressure. The resistance is provided by plasma proteins and other substances in the blood.

The blood pressure changes in response to changes in cardiac output. In other words, as the cardiac output increases, so does the blood pressure. If the cardiac output decreases, so does the blood pressure. If either the stroke volume or heart rate increases, so does the cardiac output and, as a result, the blood pressure rises. Conversely, if the stroke volume or heart rate decreases, so do both the cardiac output and the blood pressure. The volume of blood pumped out from the ventricle with each contraction is called the stroke volume and this equals around 70 mL for an adult at rest.

The control of blood pressure

Blood pressure is controlled and regulated by a number of factors, such as baroreceptors, chemoreceptors, hypothalamus, circulating hormones and the renin-angiotensin system.

Baroreceptors

These are located in the arch of the aorta and the carotid sinus, and are sensitive to pressure changes within the blood vessel. When the blood pressure increases, signals are sent to the cardioregulatory centre (CRC) in the brainstem (medulla oblongata) (Figure 21.1). The cardioregulatory centre increases the parasympathetic activity to the heart, reducing heart rate and inhibiting sympathetic activity to the blood vessels; this causes vasodilation, reducing blood pressure. However, if the blood pressure falls, then the CRC increases the sympathetic activity to the heart and blood vessels, thus increasing heart rate and vasoconstriction, resulting in increased blood pressure.

Chemoreceptors

Chemoreceptors are found close to the carotid and aortic baroreceptors in small structures called carotid bodies and aortic bodies. They are sensitive to any change in the chemical composition of the blood, such as a decrease in oxygen level and pH of the blood or an increase in the carbon dioxide level. These receptors send impulses to the cardiovascular centre which in turn increases the sympathetic stimulation to the blood vessels, causing an increase in blood pressure. Chemoreceptors also stimulate the respiratory centres in the brain to increase the rate of respiration.

Circulating hormones

Hormones, for example, antidiuretic (ADH) and atrial natriuretic peptide (ANP), help in controlling circulating blood volume by fluid and electrolyte regulation, thus affecting the blood pressure. The hormones are released when the body is dehydrated and this causes the kidneys to conserve water, thus concentrating the urine and reducing its volume. At high concentrations, blood pressure is raised, stimulating moderate vasoconstriction.

Atrial natriuretic peptide is a powerful vasodilator, and a protein (polypeptide) hormone that is secreted by heart muscle cells. It is released by the atria of the heart. ANP acts to reduce water, sodium and adipose levels in the circulatory system, thereby reducing blood pressure.

Renin-angiotensin system

This system helps to maintain blood pressure through its action on vasoconstriction by generating angiotensin II. When blood volume is low, juxtaglomerular cells located in the kidneys secrete renin directly into the circulation. Plasma renin then carries out the conversion of angiotensinogen released by the liver to angiotensin I. Angiotensin I is subsequently converted to angiotensin II by the angiotensin converting enzyme in the lungs. Angiotensin II is a potent vasoactive peptide that causes blood vessels to constrict, resulting in increased blood pressure.

Angiotensin II stimulates the release of the hormone aldosterone in the adrenal glands, which causes the renal tubules to retain sodium and water and excrete potassium. Together, angiotensin II and aldosterone work to raise blood volume, blood pressure and sodium levels in the blood to restore the balance of sodium, potassium and fluids. If the renin-angiotensin system becomes overactive, consistently high blood pressure results.

Hypothalamus

The hypothalamus, located in the brain, responds to stimuli such as emotion, pain and anger, stimulating sympathetic nervous activity and affecting blood pressure.

Taking a blood pressure measurement

The blood pressure is measured using a sphygmomanometer (electronic, digital or aneroid), which is a non-invasive method of monitoring a patient's blood pressure (Figure 21.2). It may be used as a diagnostic test with patients who have arterial blood pressure problems. It can be recorded with the patient sitting comfortably in a chair or lying in bed. Taking and recording blood pressure is a skill that health and care professionals need to be competent in.

Ambulatory blood pressure monitoring is also sometimes used to check how well medicines used to treat hypertension are working.

Clinical practice point

Ambulatory blood pressure monitoring (ABPM) is undertaken with a special device that consists of a blood pressure cuff that is worn on the arm and is attached to a small recording device that is worn on a belt. The ABPM device is worn for either 24 or 48 hours and records the blood pressure periodically (usually at 15-minute or 30-minute intervals) throughout that period, during routine daily activities and while the person is sleeping but the person must avoid getting the equipment wet. The technique most commonly used for evaluating the results of ABPM is to average a person's systolic and diastolic blood pressures for a full 24-hour period and also for the hours that the person is awake and asleep.

22 The lymphatic circulation

Figure 22.1 The lymphatic system and organs.

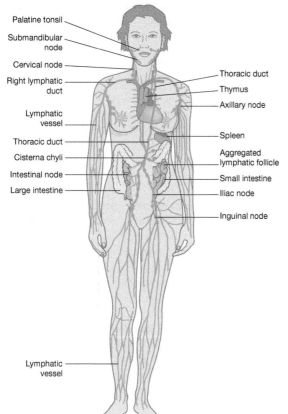

- Palatine tonsil
- Submandibular node
- Cervical node
- Right lymphatic duct
- Lymphatic vessel
- Thoracic duct
- Cisterna chyli
- Intestinal node
- Large intestine
- Thoracic duct
- Thymus
- Axillary node
- Spleen
- Aggregated lymphatic follicle
- Small intestine
- Iliac node
- Inguinal node
- Lymphatic vessel

Figure 22.2 The lymphatic capillaries.

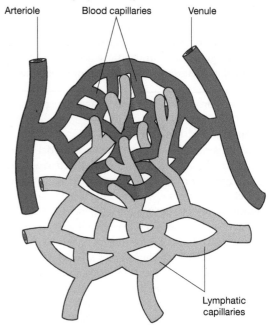

- Arteriole
- Blood capillaries
- Venule
- Lymphatic capillaries

Source: Peate I & Nair M. Fundamentals of Anatomy and Physiology for Student Nurses (2011).

Figure 22.3 Lymph node.

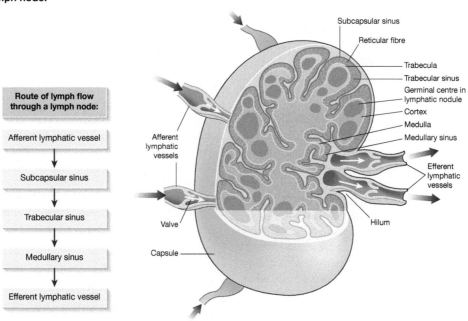

Route of lymph flow through a lymph node:

Afferent lymphatic vessel

↓

Subcapsular sinus

↓

Trabecular sinus

↓

Medullary sinus

↓

Efferent lymphatic vessel

- Subcapsular sinus
- Reticular fibre
- Trabecula
- Trabecular sinus
- Germinal centre in lymphatic nodule
- Cortex
- Medulla
- Medullary sinus
- Efferent lymphatic vessels
- Hilum
- Afferent lymphatic vessels
- Valve
- Capsule

Source: Peate I & Nair M. Fundamentals of Anatomy and Physiology for Student Nurses (2011).

Anatomy and Physiology for Nursing and Healthcare Students at a Glance, Second Edition. Ian Peate.
© 2022 John Wiley & Sons Ltd. Published 2022 by John Wiley & Sons Ltd.
Companion website: www.wiley.com/go/peate/anatomyandphysiology

Functions of the lymphatic system

The functions of the lymphatic system are to destroy pathogens and filter waste, dead blood cells, cancer cells and toxins before returning useful substances to the circulation. It also delivers oxygen, nutrients and hormones from the blood to the cells.

The lymphatic system

The lymphatic system is a network of tissues and organs that primarily consists of lymph vessels, lymph nodes and lymph. The tonsils, adenoids, spleen and thymus are all part of this system (Figure 22.1). There are 600–700 lymph nodes in the body that are responsible for filtering the lymph before it is returned to the circulatory system.

The spleen, which is largest of the lymphatic organs, is located on the left side of the body just above the left kidney. Humans can live without a spleen, although people who have had a splenectomy as a result of disease or injury are more prone to infections.

The thymus, which stores immature lymphocytes and prepares them to become active T cells, is located in the chest just above the heart.

The tonsils are large clusters of lymphatic cells found in the pharynx. Although tonsillectomies occur much less frequently today than they did in the 1950s, for example, it is still among the most common of surgical procedures performed today and typically follows frequent throat infections.

Lymphatic capillaries (Figure 22.2) differ from blood capillaries in that they originate as pockets rather than forming continuous vessels, they have larger diameters with thinner walls and have an irregular outline.

Lymph

Lymph is a clear, colourless fluid that is found inside the lymphatic capillaries and has a similar composition to plasma. Lymph is the ultra-filtrate of the blood which occurs at the capillary ends of the blood vessels.

This fluid contains white blood cells (lymphocytes), along with a small concentration of red blood cells and proteins. It circulates freely through the body, bathing the cells in needed nutrients and oxygen while it collects harmful materials for disposal. Lymph may pick up bacteria and bring them to lymph nodes where they are destroyed.

Lymph nodes

Lymph nodes are bean-shaped organs scattered along the lymphatic vessels. These nodes are found in the largest concentrations at the neck, axillae, thorax, abdomen and groin (Figure 22.3) and lesser concentrations are found behind the elbows and knees.

Lymph vessels route the fluid through nodes located throughout the body. Lymph nodes are small structures that work as filters for harmful substances. They contain immune cells that can attack and destroy harmful microbes in the lymph fluid to help fight infection. Each lymph node filters fluid and substances picked up by the vessels that lead to it. Lymph fluid from the fingers, for instance, works its way toward the chest, joining fluid from the arm. This fluid may filter through lymph nodes at the elbow or those in the axillae. Fluid from the head, scalp and face flows down through lymph nodes located in the neck. At the end of the circulation, useful substances, for example protein and salts, are returned to the general circulation.

Lymphatic organs

The organs of the lymphatic system are depicted in Figure 22.1.

Spleen

The spleen is an organ about the size of a clenched fist which is found on the left-hand side of the upper abdomen. Its main functions are to filter the blood, create new blood cells and store platelets. It is also a key part of the body's immune system.

The spleen contains two main types of tissue: white pulp and red pulp. White pulp is lymphatic tissue (material which is part of the immune system) mainly made up of white blood cells. Red pulp is made up of venous sinuses (blood-filled cavities) and splenic cords. Splenic cords are special tissues which contain different types of red and white blood cells.

Blood flows into the spleen where it enters the white pulp. Here, white blood cells called B and T cells screen the blood. T cells help to recognise invading pathogens, for example bacteria and viruses that might cause illness, and then destroy them. B cells make antibodies that help to stop infections from proliferating.

Blood also enters the red pulp where the damaged red blood cells are removed and stores platelets. In the fetus, red pulp produces new red blood cells but this function ceases after birth.

Thymus gland

The thymus is a pinkish-grey colour, soft and lobulated on its surfaces. At birth it is about 5 cm in length, 4 cm in breadth and about 6 mm in thickness. The thymus gland consists of two lobes joined by connective tissue and each lobe is covered by an outer cortex and an inner portion known as the medulla.

The thymus is an important part of children's immune systems. It grows larger until puberty and then begins to shrink.

The gland produces thymosins, which are hormones that stimulate the development of antibodies. The thymus also produces T lymphocytes which are white blood cells that fight infections and destroy abnormal cells. Once matured, these T lymphocytes, or T cells, circulate through the bloodstream and collect in the lymph organs such as the spleen and lymph nodes, for future use.

Clinical practice point

An enlarged spleen (splenomegaly). The spleen can become enlarged as a result of an infection or injury and also as a result of a health condition, such as cirrhosis, leukaemia or rheumatoid arthritis. An enlarged spleen does not always cause symptoms. Symptoms may include feeling full very quickly after eating, feeling discomfort or pain behind the left ribs, anaemia and fatigue, recurrent infections, a tendency to bleed easily. The spleen is not usually removed (splenectomy) if it is just enlarged. Treatment for any underlying condition is provided and the spleen will be monitored. If there is an infection antibiotics may be provided. The person is advised to avoid contact sports for a while, they are at greater risk of rupturing the spleen while it is enlarged. Surgery is only required if the enlarged spleen is causing serious complications or the cause cannot be found.

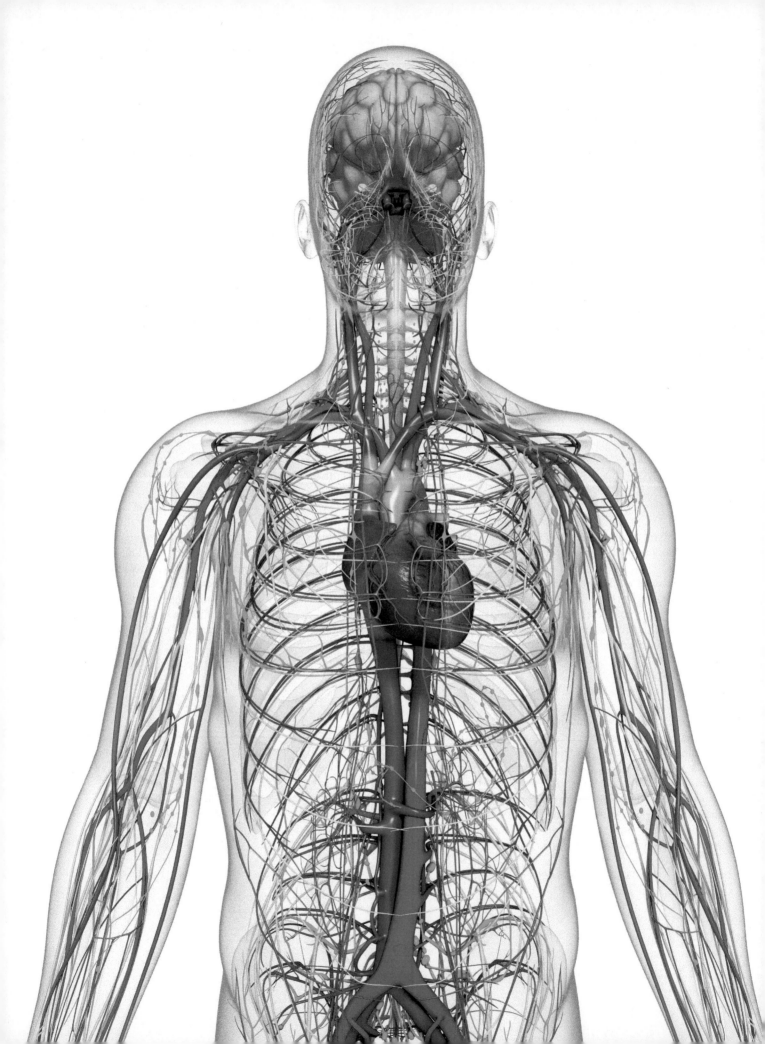

The respiratory system

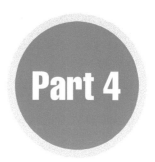

Part 4

Chapters

23 The respiratory tract

Figure 23.1 The respiratory organs.

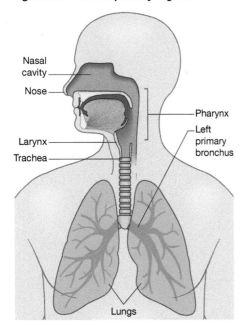

Source: Peate I, Wild K & Nair M (eds). Nursing Practice: Knowledge and Care (2014).

Figure 23.2 Detailed structures of the respiratory tract.

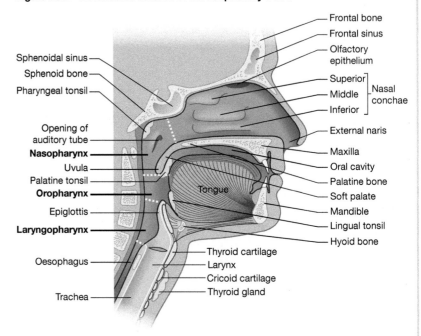

Source: Peate I, Wild K & Nair M (eds). Nursing Practice: Knowledge and Care (2014).

Figure 23.3 The lower respiratory tract.

Branching of bronchial tree

- Trachea
- Primary bronchi
- Secondary bronchi
- Tertiary bronchi
- Bronchioles
- Terminal bronchioles

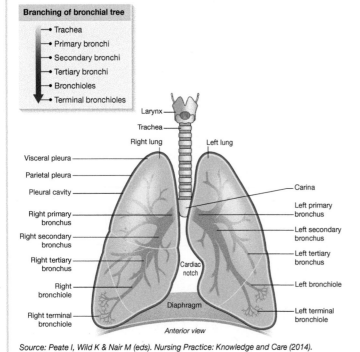

Anterior view

Source: Peate I, Wild K & Nair M (eds). Nursing Practice: Knowledge and Care (2014).

Figure 23.4 Bronchial tree.

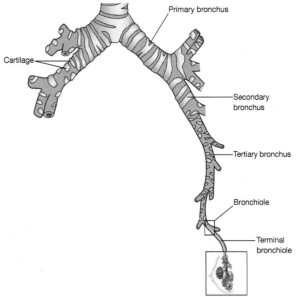

Source: Peate I & Nair M. Fundamentals of Anatomy and Physiology for Student Nurses (2011).

Anatomy and Physiology for Nursing and Healthcare Students at a Glance, Second Edition. Ian Peate.
© 2022 John Wiley & Sons Ltd. Published 2022 by John Wiley & Sons Ltd.
Companion website: www.wiley.com/go/peate/anatomyandphysiology

The respiratory tract is responsible for gaseous exchange between the circulatory system and the atmosphere. Air is taken in via the upper airways (the nasal cavity, pharynx and larynx), passed through the lower airways (trachea, primary bronchi and bronchial tree) and into the small bronchioles and alveoli within the lung tissue. Structurally, the respiratory tract is divided into the upper and lower respiratory tracts/systems. The upper respiratory system comprises the nasal cavity, oral cavity, pharynx and their associated structures. The lower respiratory system consists of the trachea, bronchi, bronchioles and alveoli. See Figure 23.1 the respiratory organs.

Upper respiratory tract

The mouth, nose, nasal cavity and pharynx are the organs of the upper respiratory tract. The functions of this section of the system are to warm, filter and moisten the inhaled air. The nasal cavity is divided into two equal sections by the nasal septum, a structure formed out of the ethmoid bones and the vomer of the skull. The space where air enters the nasal cavity, just inside the nostrils, is referred to as the vestibule.

The nasal cavities are subdivided into three air passageways, the meatuses, which are formed by three shelf-like projections called the superior, middle and inferior conchae or turbinates. The incoming air bounces off the conchal surface and swirls. Small particles in the air are then trapped in the mucosa of the nasal cavity (Figure 23.2).

The pharynx is a chamber shared by the digestive and respiratory systems. The pharynx connects the nasal and oral cavity with the larynx. The pharynx is divided into three regions called the nasopharynx, the oropharynx and the laryngopharynx. The nasopharynx sits behind the nasal cavity and contains two openings that lead to the auditory (eustachian) tubes.

Both the oropharynx and the laryngopharynx are passageways for food and drink as well as air and they are lined with non-keratinised stratified squamous epithelium.

Lower respiratory tract

The lower respiratory tract includes the larynx, the trachea, the right and left primary bronchi and all the constituents of both lungs (Figure 23.3). The lungs are two cone-shaped organs which almost fill the thorax. They are protected by a framework of bones, the thoracic cage, which consists of the ribs, sternum (breastbone) and vertebrae (spine). The air passages are lined with mucous membrane composed mainly of ciliated epithelium. Cilia constantly clean the tract and transport foreign matter upwards for swallowing or expectoration.

Larynx

The larynx is made up of nine pieces of cartilage tissue – three single pieces and three pairs. The single pieces of cartilage are the thyroid, epiglottis and cricoid cartilage. The thyroid cartilage is more commonly known as the Adam's apple and, together with the cricoid cartilage, it protects the vocal cords. The epiglottis is a leaf-shaped piece of elastic cartilage attached to the top of the larynx. Its function is to protect the airway from food and fluids. On swallowing, the epiglottis blocks entry to the larynx and food and liquids are diverted towards the oesophagus, which sits nearby.

Trachea

The trachea (windpipe) extends from the laryngopharynx at the level of the cricoid cartilage at the top to the carina (also known as the tracheal bifurcation). The trachea contains 15–20 C-shaped cartilage rings that reinforce and protect the trachea to prevent it from collapse or overexpansion as pressure changes within the respiratory system. The carina is a ridge-shaped structure at the level of T6 or T7. It has sensory nerve endings which cause coughing if food or fluids are inhaled accidentally.

Bronchi and bronchioles

The trachea (windpipe) is divided into two main bronchi (also called mainstem bronchi), the left and the right, at the level of the sternal angle and the fifth thoracic vertebra or up to two vertebrae higher or lower, depending on breathing, at the anatomical point known as the carina.

The right main bronchus is more vertical, wider and shorter, and this subdivides into three lobar bronchi; the left main bronchus divides into two. The segmental bronchi divide into many primary bronchioles which divide into terminal bronchioles, each of which then gives rise to several respiratory bronchioles, which go on to divide into and terminate in tiny air sacs called alveoli (Figure 23.4).

The lungs

The lungs are divided into distinct regions called lobes. There are three lobes in the right lung and two in the left. Each lung is surrounded by two thin protective membranes known as the parietal and visceral pleura. The parietal pleura lines the wall of the thorax whereas the visceral pleura covers the lungs themselves. The space between the two pleura, the pleural space, is very small and contains a thin film of lubricating pleural fluid. This helps to reduce friction between the two pleura, permitting both layers to slide over one another during breathing. The fluid also helps the visceral and parietal pleura to adhere to each other.

Blood supply

The conduction and respiratory regions of the lungs receive blood from different arteries. The conduction region of the lungs receives oxygenated blood from capillaries that stem from the bronchial arteries, which originate from the aorta. Some of the bronchial arteries are connected to the pulmonary arteries but the majority of blood returns to the heart via the pulmonary or bronchial veins.

Clinical practice point

Measuring the peak expiratory flow rate is a non-invasive, uncomplicated and useful clinical investigation that can be used to identify variations in a person's respiratory effort over time. The peak expiratory flow rate is often used for the diagnosis, monitoring and assessment of the severity of respiratory compromise, particularly in those with asthma. The healthcare provider can encourage improvements in care by providing the person with education on the correct technique and by accurate assessment and recording of the peak expiratory flow rate. The healthcare worker should advise the patient on the action to be taken if differences between readings occur when the person is monitoring their health at home.

24 Pulmonary ventilation

Figure 24.1 Boyle's Law.

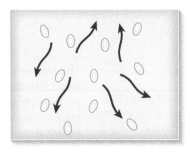

In larger volumes gases
exert less pressure

In smaller volumes gases
exert more pressure

Source: Peate I & Nair M. Fundamentals of Anatomy and Physiology for Student Nurses (2011).

Figure 24.2 Inspiration and expiration.

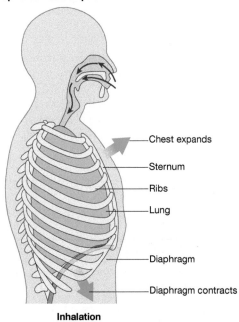

Chest expands

Sternum

Ribs

Lung

Diaphragm

Diaphragm contracts

Inhalation

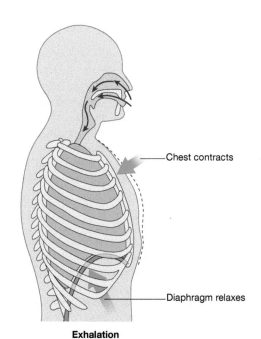

Chest contracts

Diaphragm relaxes

Exhalation

Source: Peate I & Nair M. Fundamentals of Anatomy and Physiology for Student Nurses (2011).

Anatomy and Physiology for Nursing and Healthcare Students at a Glance, Second Edition. Ian Peate.
© 2022 John Wiley & Sons Ltd. Published 2022 by John Wiley & Sons Ltd.
Companion website: www.wiley.com/go/peate/anatomyandphysiology

Breathing

Pulmonary ventilation involves the physical movement of air in and out of the lungs. The primary function of pulmonary ventilation is to maintain adequate alveolar ventilation. This prevents the build-up of carbon dioxide in the alveoli and achieves a constant supply of oxygen to the tissues.

Air flows between the atmosphere and the alveoli of the lungs as a result of a pressure difference created by the contraction and relaxation of the respiratory muscles. The rate of air flow and the effort needed for breathing are influenced by the alveoli surface tension and integrity of the lungs.

Inspiration

Breathing in is called inhalation. Just before breathing in (inhalation), the pressure in the lungs equals the atmospheric pressure (760 mmHg or 101.33 kilopascals [kPa]). Thus, for air to flow into the lungs, the pressure inside the alveoli has to be lower than the atmosphere. This is achieved by increasing the volume of the lungs.

During inspiration, the thorax expands and intrapulmonary pressure falls below atmospheric pressure. Because intrapulmonary pressure is now less than atmospheric pressure, the air will naturally enter the lungs until the pressure difference no longer exists. This phenomenon is explained by Boyle's Law (Figure 24.1) and Dalton's Law. Gases exert pressure and Boyle's Law states that the amount of pressure exerted is inversely proportional to the size of its container.

Dalton's Law states that in a mixture of gases, each gas will exert its own individual pressure proportional to its size. For example, atmospheric air contains a mixture of gases. Each individual gas will exert its own pressure dependent upon its quantity. Nitrogen, for example, will exert the greatest pressure as this is the most abundant gas. Collectively, all the gases in the atmosphere exert a pressure, atmospheric pressure, which is 101.33 kPa at sea level. On inhalation, the thorax expands and intrapulmonary pressure falls below 101.33 kPa and as a result, air enters the lungs.

A range of respiratory muscles are used to achieve thoracic expansion during the process of inspiration. The major muscles of inspiration are the diaphragm and external intercostal muscles. The diaphragm is a dome-shaped skeletal muscle located beneath the lungs at the base of the thorax. There are 11 external intercostal muscles, which sit in the intercostal spaces, between the ribs. During inspiration, the diaphragm contracts downwards, pulling the lungs with it (Figure 24.2). Simultaneously, the external intercostal muscles will pull the rib cage outwards and upwards. The thorax is now bigger than before and intrapulmonary pressure is reduced below atmospheric pressure as a result. The most important muscle of inspiration is the diaphragm; 75% of the air that enters the lungs is as a result of diaphragmatic contraction.

Exhalation

Breathing out (exhalation) is also as a result of a pressure gradient but it is converse to inhalation; that is, the pressure in the lungs is greater than in the atmosphere. At rest, normal exhalation is a passive process as there are no skeletal muscles involved. The process results from elastic recoil of the chest walls and the lungs (see Figure 24.2).

Exhalation increases during certain activities, for example exercise. During exercise, the muscles of exhalation, which are the abdominals and intercostal muscles, contract thus increasing the abdominal and thoracic region.

As the abdominal muscle contracts, the inferior ribs move downwards and compress the abdominal viscera, and the diaphragm moves upwards (see Figure 24.2).

Factors affecting pulmonary ventilation

Surface tension of alveolar fluid

Surface tension is provided by a fluid called surfactant, which is a mixture of phospholipids and lipoproteins. During inhalation, the surface tension has to be overcome so as to expand the lungs. It also aids in the lungs' elastic recoil.

Airway resistance

The flow of air through airway passages depends on the resistance and pressure difference. The walls of the airways offer some resistance to the flow of air into and out of the lungs. During inspiration, the bronchioles dilate as their walls are pulled in all directions. The diameter of the airway passage is also dependent on the smooth muscles. Stimulation from the sympathetic nerve fibres will cause the smooth muscles to relax and this results in bronchodilation and decreased resistance.

Compliance of the lungs

Compliance means the effort required for lung and chest expansion. The higher the compliance, the less effort is needed in chest and lung expansion, and low compliance means that more effort is needed. In the lungs, there are two factors that play a part in compliance: surface tension and elasticity.

Normal lungs have a high compliance and expand easily because the elastic fibres stretch readily and surfactant in the lungs reduces surface tension. In pulmonary diseases, for example emphysema, there is decreased compliance due to loss of elastic fibres of the alveolar walls.

Lung volumes

A healthy adult at rest will normally have a respiratory rate of 12–18 breaths per minute and with each respiration, 500 mL of air is moved in or out of the lungs. The volume of air in one breath is known as tidal volume. By taking a deep breath, the tidal volume can be increased above 500 mL (inspiratory reserve volume). In an adult male, this could be up to 3100 mL and in females it is approximately 1900 mL.

Clinical practice point

Spirometry is a simple test that is used to diagnose and monitor certain lung conditions by measuring how much air a person can breathe out in one forced breath. It is carried out using a device called a spirometer, which is a small machine attached by a cable to a mouthpiece. Spirometry can be undertaken by a competent healthcare professional at a GP surgery, or it can be carried out during a visit to a hospital or clinic. Conditions that can be detected and monitored using spirometry include asthma, chronic obstructive pulmonary disease, cystic fibrosis and pulmonary fibrosis.

25 Control of breathing

Figure 25.1   The respiratory centre.

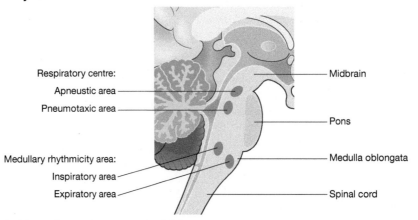

Respiratory centre:
Apneustic area
Pneumotaxic area

Medullary rhythmicity area:
Inspiratory area
Expiratory area

Midbrain

Pons

Medulla oblongata

Spinal cord

Source: Peate I, Wild K & Nair M (eds). Nursing Practice: Knowledge and Care (2014).

Figure 25.2   Peripheral chemoreceptors.

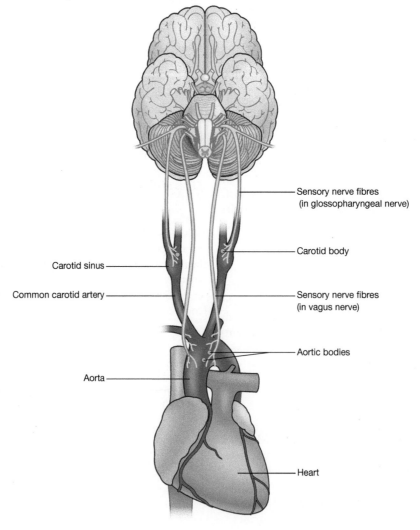

Sensory nerve fibres
(in glossopharyngeal nerve)

Carotid body

Carotid sinus

Common carotid artery

Sensory nerve fibres
(in vagus nerve)

Aortic bodies

Aorta

Heart

There is an area in the brainstem called the respiratory centre. This consists of the medullary rhythmicity area, which controls the basic rhythm of respiration, the pneumotaxic area, which helps co-ordinate the transition between inspiration and expiration, and the apneustic area, which also co-ordinates the transition between inspiration and expiration.

Medullary rhythmic area

The function of the medullary rhythmic area is to control the respiratory rhythm. There are inspiratory and expiratory areas located within the medullary rhythmicity area (Figure 25.1). During quiet breathing, inhalation is about 2 seconds while expiration is around 3 seconds. Impulses from the inspiratory area maintain this rhythm. When the inspiratory area is active, then the expiratory area is inactive.

However, during forceful breathing the expiratory area is stimulated by nerves from the inspiratory area. Stimulation by the expiratory area causes the intercostal muscles and abdominals to contract, which causes a decrease in the thoracic cavity and forceful exhalation.

Pneumotaxic area

The pneumotaxic area (see Figure 25.1) is in the pons and is important for regulating the amount of air taken in with each breath. However, the inspiratory musculature is controlled by the dorsal respiratory group. This is where the pneumotaxic area comes into play. The pneumotaxic area alters the bursting pattern of the dorsal respiratory group. When we need to breathe faster, the pneumotaxic area tells the dorsal respiratory group to speed it up. When we need to take longer breaths, the pneumotaxic area tells the dorsal respiratory group to prolong its bursts. All the information from the body that feeds into the control of our breathing converges in the pneumotaxic area, so that it can properly adjust our breathing.

Apneustic area

Another part of the brain that co-ordinates transition between inhalation and exhalation is the apneustic area, situated in the lower pons (see Figure 25.1). This area sends signals to the inspiratory area that then activate and prolong inhalation, resulting in long, deep inhalation. When the pneumotaxic area is active, it will override the signals from the apneustic area.

Central chemoreceptors

These areas are found in the brainstem and contain neurons, central chemoreceptors, that detect changes in carbon dioxide levels. The way they do this is somewhat indirect. When the carbon dioxide levels rise, that means that the respiration rate has to increase, in order to get rid of the carbon dioxide and take in more oxygen. Carbon dioxide does not tend to remain as carbon dioxide in water. Instead, it changes into a bicarbonate ion, producing hydrogen ions as a by-product of this conversion.

In blood, when carbon dioxide is converted into bicarbonate ions, the hydrogen ions are not a problem because they immediately associate with haemoglobin (the globin acts to buffer the hydrogen ions). However, in the brain, in the chemosensitive areas, there is no haemoglobin. The cerebrospinal fluid of the brain does not have proteins to buffer the hydrogen ions so when levels of carbon dioxide in the brain begin to increase, much of it is converted into bicarbonate ions and hydrogen ions. The central chemoreceptors are sensitive to hydrogen ion levels so they indirectly recognise the increase in carbon dioxide levels.

However, a change in plasma pH alone will not stimulate central chemoreceptors as hydrogen ions are not able to diffuse across the blood–brain barrier into the CSF. Only carbon dioxide levels affect this as it can diffuse across, reacting with water to form carbonic acid, and as such will result in a decrease in the pH. Central chemoreception remains in this way distinct from peripheral chemoreceptors.

Peripheral chemoreceptors

The peripheral chemoreceptors are not quite as important as the central chemoreceptors. Where the common carotid artery branches into the internal and external carotid arteries, there is a small swelling (Figure 25.2). This is the carotid sinus and it contains regions called carotid bodies. The aorta contains regions called aortic bodies. These regions contain the peripheral chemoreceptors, which detect oxygen levels directly. Exactly how these neurons can be sensitive to oxygen is not the issue here, but instead, it is interesting to note that these neurons can only detect large decreases in oxygen levels so they are only activated when oxygen levels drop to very low, life-threatening degrees.

Each carotid body is a few millimetres in size and has the distinction of having the highest blood flow per tissue weight of any organ in the body. Afferent nerve fibres join with the sinus nerve before entering the glossopharyngeal nerve. A decrease in carotid body blood flow results in cellular hypoxia, hypercapnia and decreased pH that lead to an increase in receptor stimulation.

Inflation reflex

This reflex, like most, is a kind of negative feedback. As the lungs expand, sensory neurons detect lung stretching; they are called stretch receptors, but they are not at all like the stretch receptors in muscle. The more these neurons are active, the more they send signals into the pneumotaxic area and tell it to end this round of inspiration. This then prevents the lungs from ever overinflating.

Other influences on respiration

Limbic system

This system can increase the rate and depth of ventilation in times of stress through inspiratory area stimulation.

Temperature

An increase or decrease in body temperature, for example pyrexia and hypothermia, can increase or decrease the respiration rate.

Pain

Sudden severe pain can cause a brief period of apnoea while a prolonged somatic pain increases the respiration rate.

Irritation of the airways

Cessation of breathing can result from physical or chemical irritation of the pharynx. This is followed by coughing and sneezing.

Clinical practice point

Hyperventilation occurs when a person overbreathes, i.e. if they breathe in excess of the body's needs. Acute hyperventilation is common at times of stress or excitement when the breathing rate increases. This may cause feelings of anxiety and physical symptoms such as breathlessness or palpitations. Chronic hyperventilation happens if the breathing pattern does not return to normal after an acute event, and chronic changes in breathing pattern may occur. It may produce a variety of symptoms that may be intermittent or continuous. Minor stresses may trigger these changes.

26 Gas exchange

Figure 26.1   External respiration.

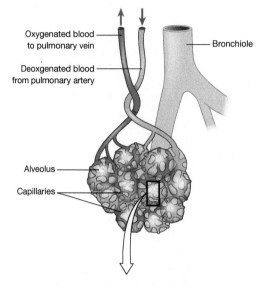

Oxygenated blood
to pulmonary vein

Deoxgenated blood
from pulmonary artery

Bronchiole

Alveolus

Capillaries

Figure 26.2   Gas exchange in the lungs.

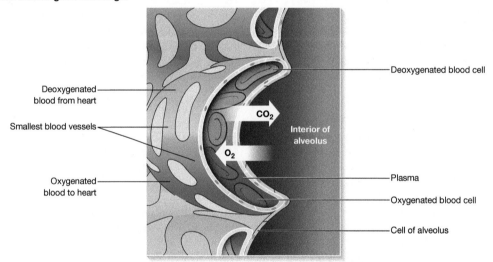

Deoxygenated
blood from heart

Smallest blood vessels

Oxygenated
blood to heart

Deoxygenated blood cell

CO_2

Interior of
alveolus

O_2

Plasma

Oxygenated blood cell

Cell of alveolus

Figure 26.3   Internal respiration.

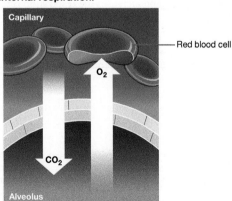

Capillary

Red blood cell

O_2

CO_2

Alveolus

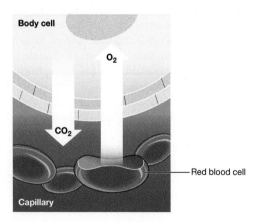

Body cell

O_2

CO_2

Red blood cell

Capillary

Anatomy and Physiology for Nursing and Healthcare Students at a Glance, Second Edition. Ian Peate.
© 2022 John Wiley & Sons Ltd. Published 2022 by John Wiley & Sons Ltd.
Companion website: www.wiley.com/go/peate/anatomyandphysiology

External respiration

External respiration (pulmonary gas exchange) is the diffusion of oxygen from the alveolar sac to the lung capillaries and the diffusion of carbon dioxide from the lung capillaries to the alveolar sac to be exhaled.

External respiration only occurs beyond the respiratory bronchioles. For this reason, the end portion of the bronchial tree is called the respiratory zone. The remainder of the bronchial tree from the trachea down to the terminal bronchioles is the conducting zone. External respiration is the diffusion of oxygen from the alveoli into the pulmonary circulation (blood flow through the lungs) and the diffusion of carbon dioxide in the opposite direction (Figure 26.1). Diffusion occurs because gas molecules always move from areas of high concentration to areas of low concentration.

Exchange of gases in the lungs

Exchange of gases in the lungs takes place between alveolar air and the blood flowing through the lung capillaries (Figure 26.2). Before oxygen can enter the internal environment and before carbon dioxide can leave it, they must cross the capillary and alveolar membranes. Oxygen enters the blood from the alveolar sac because the partial pressure of oxygen (PO_2) of alveolar air is greater than the PO_2 of incoming blood. Simultaneously, carbon dioxide molecules leave the blood by diffusing down the carbon dioxide pressure gradient out into the alveolar sac. The partial pressure of carbon dioxide (PcO_2) of venous blood is much higher than the PcO_2 of alveolar air.

Fick's Law

Fick's Law describes the movement of gases (oxygen and carbon dioxide) across the respiratory membrane of the alveoli. This is explained by the following formula:

$$J = \left(S/wt_{mol} \right) \times A \times \Delta C / t$$

J = Rate of diffusion
S/wt_{mol} = Solubility/molecular weight
A = Surface area
ΔC = Concentration difference
t = Membrane thickness

It takes around 0.25 seconds for an oxygen molecule to diffuse from the alveoli into pulmonary circulation. However, there are various influencing factors that determine the rate at which oxygen and carbon dioxide diffuse between alveoli and pulmonary circulation. Thus it could be said that the diffusion of gases is more efficient if the surface area is large, if the thickness of the membrane is small, the solubility of gas is high and the partial pressure gradient is high.

Internal respiration

Internal respiration describes the exchange of oxygen and carbon dioxide between blood and tissue cells (Figure 26.3), a phenomenon governed by the same principles as external respiration. Cells utilise oxygen when manufacturing their prime energy source, adenosine triphosphate (ATP). In addition to ATP, cells also produce water and carbon dioxide. Because cells are continually using oxygen, its concentration within the tissues is always lower than within blood. Likewise, the continual use of oxygen ensures that the level of carbon dioxide within a tissue is always higher than within blood. As blood flows through the capillaries, oxygen and carbon dioxide follow their pressure gradients and continually diffuse between blood and tissue.

Blood flowing away from the tissues, back towards the heart, is described as being deoxygenated. In reality, if measured, the oxygen saturation of venous blood would probably be around 75%. This means that only around 25% of arterial oxygen content (CaO_2) leaves the bloodstream, leaving a plentiful supply.

Factors affecting pulmonary and systemic gas exchange

Partial pressure difference of gases

Alveolar PO_2 has got to be greater than blood PO_2 in order for oxygen to diffuse out from the alveolar sac into the lung capillaries. Certain factors, for example exercise and drugs, can affect the rate of diffusion. Morphine slows the rate of ventilation, thus affecting gas exchange in the lungs.

Surface area available for gas exchange

A pulmonary disorder can affect gas exchange. Conditions such as emphysema and carcinoma of the lungs can result in poor ventilation. In emphysema, alveolar walls are destroyed and there are few functional alveolar sacs available for gas exchange.

Diffusion difference

Usually, gas exchange within the lungs occurs without any problem as the alveolar and lung capillaries are in close proximity. However, when the person experiences conditions such as pulmonary oedema, gas exchange is affected. Fluid fills the alveolar sac, making the distance greater and thus slowing down the gas exchange.

Solubility of gases

Oxygen has a lower molecular weight than carbon dioxide and thus diffuses at a greater rate. However, carbon dioxide is much more soluble in fluid than oxygen, so the net outward movement of carbon dioxide is far greater than the net inward movement of oxygen.

Transport of gases

Both oxygen and carbon dioxide are transported from the lungs to the body tissues in blood. Both gases travel in blood plasma and haemoglobin, which is found within erythrocytes (red blood cells). Each erythrocyte contains approximately 280 million haemoglobin molecules and each haemoglobin molecule has the potential to carry four oxygen molecules. The delivery of oxygen, therefore, is also reliant upon the presence of an adequate supply of erythrocytes and haemoglobin (Hb).

Just like oxygen, a small amount of carbon dioxide, around 10%, is transported in plasma. Carbon dioxide is also transported attached to haemoglobin, although only around 30% is transported that way.

Clinical practice point

Lung disease can lead to severe abnormalities in blood gas composition. Because of the differences in oxygen and carbon dioxide transport, impaired oxygen exchange is far more common than impaired carbon dioxide exchange. When a person's breathing is impaired, the lungs cannot easily move oxygen into the blood and remove carbon dioxide from the blood (gas exchange is impaired). This can result in a low oxygen level (hypoxia) or high carbon dioxide level (hypercapnia), or both, in the blood. Respiratory insufficiency refers to conditions that reduce the body's ability to perform gas exchange, including chronic obstructive pulmonary disease, interstitial lung disease, neuromuscular disease and restrictive lung disease.

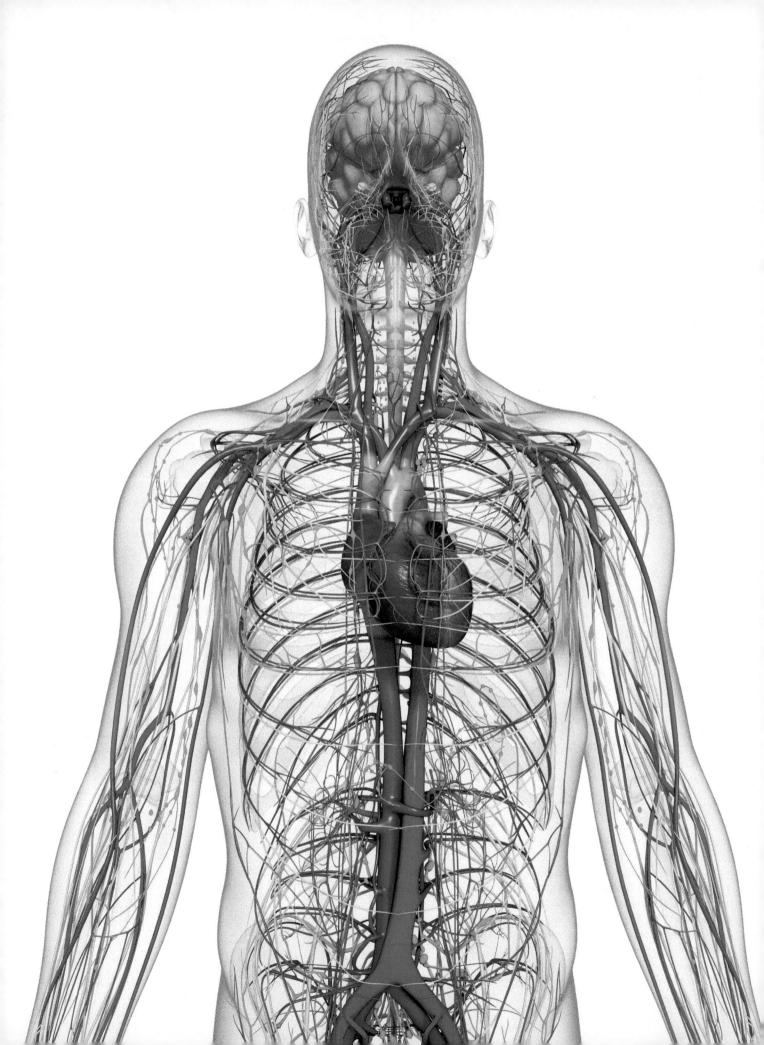

The gastrointestinal tract

Part 5

Chapters

27　The upper gastrointestinal tract

Figure 27.1　The upper and lower gastrointestinal tract.

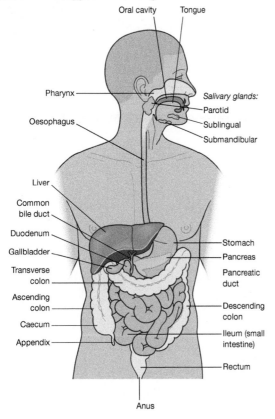

Oral cavity
Tongue
Pharynx
Oesophagus
Salivary glands:
Parotid
Sublingual
Submandibular
Liver
Common bile duct
Duodenum
Gallbladder
Transverse colon
Ascending colon
Caecum
Appendix
Anus
Stomach
Pancreas
Pancreatic duct
Descending colon
Ileum (small intestine)
Rectum

Figure 27.2　The tongue.

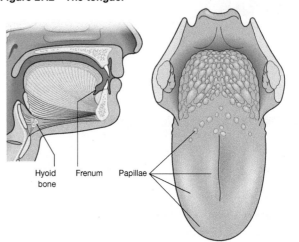

Hyoid bone
Frenum
Papillae

Figure 27.3　Swallowing action.

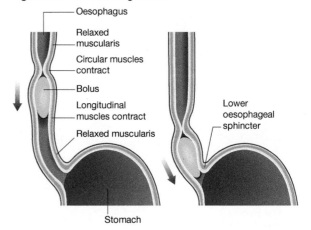

Oesophagus
Relaxed muscularis
Circular muscles contract
Bolus
Longitudinal muscles contract
Relaxed muscularis
Lower oesophageal sphincter
Stomach

Source: Peate I, Wild K & Nair M (eds). Nursing Practice: Knowledge and Care (2014).

Figure 27.4　The stomach.

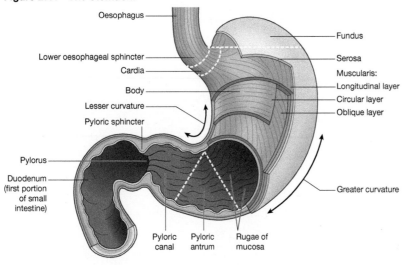

Oesophagus
Lower oesophageal sphincter
Cardia
Body
Lesser curvature
Pyloric sphincter
Pylorus
Duodenum (first portion of small intestine)
Pyloric canal
Pyloric antrum
Rugae of mucosa
Fundus
Serosa
Muscularis:
Longitudinal layer
Circular layer
Oblique layer
Greater curvature

Source: Peate I, Wild K & Nair M (eds). Nursing Practice: Knowledge and Care (2014).

Anatomy and Physiology for Nursing and Healthcare Students at a Glance, Second Edition. Ian Peate.
© 2022 John Wiley & Sons Ltd. Published 2022 by John Wiley & Sons Ltd.
Companion website: www.wiley.com/go/peate/anatomyandphysiology

The mouth (the oral cavity)

The mouth or oral cavity is where the process of digestion begins (Figure 27.1). The oral cavity is composed of several different structures. The lips and cheeks are muscular connective tissue structures, lined with mucus-secreting, stratified squamous epithelial cells providing protection against abrasion caused by wear and tear.

Lips and cheeks

The lips and cheeks move and hold the food in the mouth while the teeth tear and grind the food. This process is called mastication (chewing). The lips and cheeks are also involved in speech and facial expression.

The tongue

The tongue is a muscular organ, covered with moist, pink tissue called mucosa. The tiny bumps on the tongue are called papillae and give the tongue its rough texture. Thousands of taste buds cover the surfaces of the papillae. Taste buds are collections of nerve-like cells that connect to nerves running into the brain. The tongue is anchored to the mouth by webs of tough tissue and mucosa. The tether holding down the front of the tongue is the frenum (Figure 27.2). In the back of the mouth, the tongue is anchored into the hyoid bone. The tongue is vital for chewing and swallowing food, as well as for speech.

Palate

The palate forms the roof of the mouth and consists of two parts: the hard palate and the soft palate. The hard palate is located anteriorly and is bony. The soft palate lies posteriorly and consists of skeletal muscle and connective tissue. The palate plays a part in swallowing. The palatine tonsils lie laterally and are lymphoid tissue. The uvula is a fold of tissue hanging down from the centre of the soft palate.

Salivary glands

Saliva is produced in and secreted from salivary glands. The basic secretory units of salivary glands are clusters of cells known as acini. These cells secrete a fluid containing water, electrolytes, mucus and enzymes, all of which flow out of the acinus into collecting ducts.

Within the ducts, the composition of the secretion is altered. Much of the sodium is actively reabsorbed, potassium is secreted and large quantities of bicarbonate ions are secreted. Bicarbonate is important because it, along with phosphate, provides a critical buffer that neutralises the massive quantities of acid that are produced in the stomach.

Oesophagus

When food exits the oropharynx, it enters the oesophagus. The oesophagus extends from the laryngopharynx to the stomach. It is a thick walled structure and measures about 25 cm in length and lies in the thoracic cavity, posterior to the trachea. The function of the oesophagus is to transport substances (food bolus) from the mouth to the stomach. Thick mucus is secreted by the mucosa of the oesophagus and this aids the passage of the food bolus and protects the oesophagus from abrasion. The upper oesophageal sphincter regulates the movement of substances allowed into the oesophagus and the lower oesophageal sphincter (also known as the cardiac sphincter) regulates the movement of substances from the oesophagus to the stomach. The muscle layer of the oesophagus differs from the rest of the digestive tract as the superior portion consists of skeletal (voluntary) muscle and the inferior portion consists of smooth (involuntary) muscle. Breathing and swallowing cannot occur at the same time.

Swallowing (deglutition)

Swallowing occurs in three phases. First is the voluntary phase, where food is moved to the oropharynx by the voluntary muscle. Next is the pharyngeal phase which is under involuntary neuromuscular control. Once the food bolus encroaches on the palatoglossal folds, or anterior tonsillar pillars, the pharyngeal phase of swallowing reflexively begins.

The third phase is the oesophageal phase. Like the pharyngeal phase of swallowing, the oesophageal phase is under involuntary neuromuscular control. The outer fibres of the upper zone are arranged longitudinally while the inner fibres have a circular configuration (Figure 27.3).

Stomach

The stomach is a muscular organ, located on the left side of the upper abdomen. The stomach receives food from the oesophagus. As food reaches the end of the oesophagus, it enters the stomach through a muscular valve called the lower oesophageal sphincter (Figure 27.4).

The stomach is supplied with arterial blood from a branch of the celiac artery and venous blood leaves the stomach via the hepatic vein. The vagus nerve innervates the stomach with parasympathetic fibres that stimulate gastric motility as well as the secretion of gastric juice.

The stomach has the same four layers of tissue found in the digestive tract but there are some differences. The muscularis contains three layers of smooth muscle instead of two. It has longitudinal, circular and oblique muscle fibres. The extra muscle layer facilitates the churning, mixing and mechanical breakdown of food that occurs within the stomach as well as supporting the onward journey of the food by peristalsis.

The stomach secretes acid and enzymes that digest food. Ridges of muscle tissue called rugae line the stomach. The stomach muscles contract periodically, churning food so as to enhance digestion. The pyloric sphincter is a muscular valve that opens to permit food to pass from the stomach into the duodenum.

Clinical practice point

Nausea and vomiting are debilitating symptoms causing discomfort and distress and can have a harmful impact on a person's quality of life, as well as increasing anxiety for family members and other carers. These are two distinct symptoms. The pathophysiology of nausea and vomiting is complex; it is believed there are two main centres involved: the chemoreceptor trigger zone (CTZ) and the vomiting centre located at brainstem level. These areas are a series of interconnecting neural networks. The CTZ is stimulated by chemicals in the cerebrospinal fluid and blood and by input from vagus and vestibular nerves. It contains receptors for dopamine, serotonin, acetylcholine and opioids. The vomiting centre receives input from a wide range of sources, including the CTZ, cerebral cortex, hypothalamus, glossopharyngeal and splenic nerves, and vagus nerve, which is stimulated by activation of mechanoreceptors and serotonin receptors in the gut (the emetic pathway). It is important to understand the cause of symptoms to address the problem as effectively as possible.

28 The lower gastrointestinal tract

Figure 28.1 The small intestine.

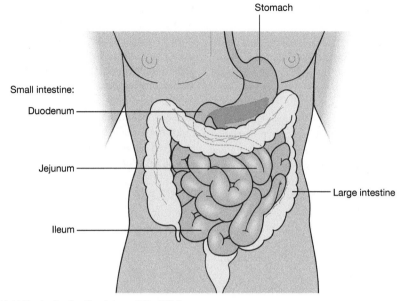

Stomach

Small intestine:

Duodenum

Jejunum

Large intestine

Ileum

Source: Peate I, Wild K & Nair M (eds). Nursing Practice: Knowledge and Care (2014).

Figure 28.2 The large intestine.

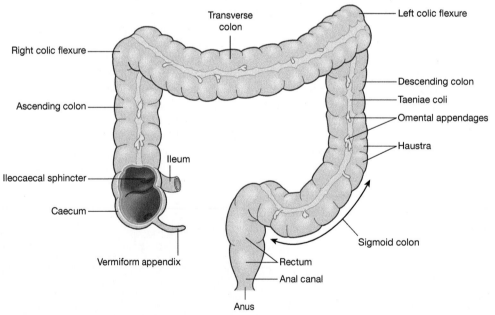

Transverse colon

Left colic flexure

Right colic flexure

Ascending colon

Descending colon

Taeniae coli

Omental appendages

Haustra

Ileum

Ileocaecal sphincter

Caecum

Sigmoid colon

Vermiform appendix

Rectum

Anal canal

Anus

Source: Peate I, Wild K & Nair M (eds). Nursing Practice: Knowledge and Care (2014).

Anatomy and Physiology for Nursing and Healthcare Students at a Glance, Second Edition. Ian Peate.
© 2022 John Wiley & Sons Ltd. Published 2022 by John Wiley & Sons Ltd.
Companion website: www.wiley.com/go/peate/anatomyandphysiology

The small intestine

The small intestine is the part of the gastrointestinal tract that follows on from the stomach and is where much of the digestion and absorption of food takes place. The small intestine consists of three sections. The first portion, the duodenum, connects to the stomach. The middle portion is the jejunum. The final section, called the ileum, attaches to the large intestine (Figure 28.1).

The small intestine receives its arterial blood supply from the superior mesenteric artery and nutrient-rich venous blood drains into the superior mesenteric vein and eventually into the hepatic portal vein toward the liver. The small intestine secretes around 1.5 L of intestinal juice daily.

Duodenum

This is a short portion of the small intestine connecting it to the stomach (see Figure 28.1). It is approximately 25 cm long, while the entire small intestine measures about 6.5 metres. This structure begins with the duodenal bulb, bordered by the pyloric sphincter that marks the lower end of the stomach, and it is connected by the ligament of Treitz to the diaphragm before leading into the next portion of the small intestine which is the jejunum.

The duodenum is primarily responsible for the breakdown of food in the small intestine, using a number of enzymes. The villi of the duodenum have a leafy-looking appearance, a histologically identifiable structure. Brunner's glands (these secrete mucus) are found in the duodenum. The duodenal wall is composed of a very thin layer of cells that form the muscularis mucosae.

The duodenum also regulates the rate of emptying of the stomach. Secretin and cholecystokinin (hormones) are released from cells in the duodenal epithelium in response to acidic and fatty stimuli present there when the pylorus opens and releases gastric chyme into the duodenum for further digestion. These cause the liver and gall bladder to release bile and the pancreas to release bicarbonate and digestive enzymes such as trypsin, lipase and amylase into the duodenum as required.

Jejunum

The section of the small intestine called the jejunum comprises the first two-fifths beyond the duodenum; it is larger, thicker-walled and more vascular and has more circular folds than the ileum.

The inner surface of the jejunum, its mucous membrane, is covered in projections called villi, which increase the surface area of tissue available to absorb nutrients from the gut contents. The epithelial cells which line these villi possess even larger numbers of microvilli.

The transportation of nutrients across epithelial cells throughout the jejunum and ileum includes the passive transport of sugar fructose and the active transport of amino acids, small peptides, vitamins and glucose. The villi in the jejunum are much longer than in the duodenum or ileum.

The jejunum contains very few Brunner's glands (found in the duodenum) or Peyer's patches (found in the ileum). However, there are a few jejunal lymph nodes suspended in its mesentery. The jejunum has many large circular folds in its submucosa called plicae circulares, which increase the surface area for nutrient absorption.

Ileum

The ileum is the final and longest segment of the small intestine. It is specifically responsible for the absorption of vitamin B12 and the reabsorption of conjugated bile salts. The ileum is about 4 metres long and extends from the jejunum (the middle section of the small intestine) to the ileocaecal valve, which empties into the colon (large intestine). The ileum is suspended from the abdominal wall by the mesentery, a fold of serous membrane.

The smooth muscle of the ileum is thinner than the walls of other parts of the intestine and its peristaltic contractions are slower. The ileum's lining is also less permeable than that of the upper small intestine. Small collections of lymphatic tissue (Peyer's patches) are embedded in the ileal wall, and specific receptors for bile salts and vitamin B12 are contained exclusively in its lining; about 90% of the conjugated bile salts in the intestinal contents is absorbed by the ileum.

The large intestine (the colon)

The large intestine, the posterior section of the intestine, consists of four regions: the cecum, colon, rectum and anus (Figure 28.2). The term 'colon' is sometimes used to refer to the entire large intestine. The large intestine is wider and shorter than the small intestine (approximately 1.5 metres in length) and it has a smooth inner wall. In the upper half of the large intestine, enzymes from the small intestine complete the digestive process and bacteria produce B vitamins (B12, thiamin and riboflavin).

The large intestine mucosa contains large numbers of goblet cells that secrete mucus to ease the passage of faeces and protect the walls of the colon. The simple columnar epithelium changes to stratified squamous epithelium at the anal canal. Anal sinuses secrete mucus in response to faecal compression. This protects the anal canal from the abrasion associated with emptying.

The food residue from the ileum is fluid when it enters the caecum and contains very few nutrients. The small intestine is responsible for some of the absorption of water but the primary function of the large intestine is to absorb water and turn the food residue into semi-solid faeces. The large intestine also absorbs some vitamins, minerals, electrolytes and drugs.

Clinical practice point

Constipation is a common condition and can occur in all age groups. Constipation can be defined as the inability to pass faeces regularly or that the person is unable to completely empty the bowel. The condition affects twice as many women as men and is also more common in older adults and during pregnancy. The severity of constipation will vary from person to person. Many people may only experience constipation for a short period but for others, constipation can be a chronic condition that may cause significant pain and discomfort and negatively affect their quality of life. It can be difficult to identify the exact cause of constipation but there are a number of things that contribute to the condition, including lack of sufficient fibre in the diet, a change in routine or lifestyle such as a change in eating habits, ignoring the urge to pass faeces, side-effects of certain medications, not drinking adequate amounts of fluids, anxiety or depression.

The liver, gall bladder and biliary tree

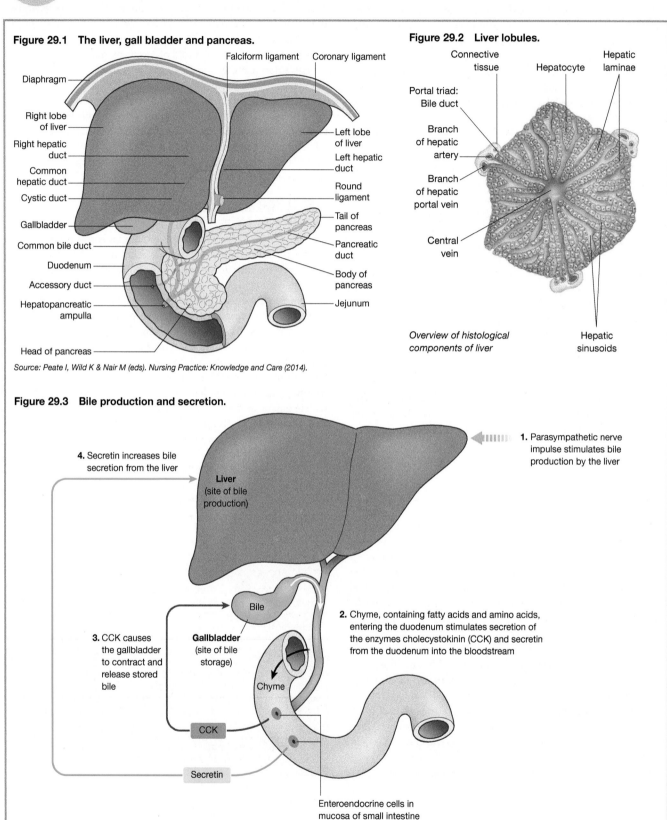

Figure 29.1   The liver, gall bladder and pancreas.

- Diaphragm
- Right lobe of liver
- Right hepatic duct
- Common hepatic duct
- Cystic duct
- Gallbladder
- Common bile duct
- Duodenum
- Accessory duct
- Hepatopancreatic ampulla
- Head of pancreas

- Falciform ligament
- Coronary ligament
- Left lobe of liver
- Left hepatic duct
- Round ligament
- Tail of pancreas
- Pancreatic duct
- Body of pancreas
- Jejunum

Source: Peate I, Wild K & Nair M (eds). Nursing Practice: Knowledge and Care (2014).

Figure 29.2   Liver lobules.

- Connective tissue
- Hepatocyte
- Hepatic laminae
- Portal triad:
  - Bile duct
  - Branch of hepatic artery
  - Branch of hepatic portal vein
- Central vein
- Hepatic sinusoids

Overview of histological components of liver

Figure 29.3   Bile production and secretion.

4. Secretin increases bile secretion from the liver

Liver (site of bile production)

1. Parasympathetic nerve impulse stimulates bile production by the liver

3. CCK causes the gallbladder to contract and release stored bile

Bile

Gallbladder (site of bile storage)

Chyme

CCK

Secretin

2. Chyme, containing fatty acids and amino acids, entering the duodenum stimulates secretion of the enzymes cholecystokinin (CCK) and secretin from the duodenum into the bloodstream

Enteroendocrine cells in mucosa of small intestine

Anatomy and Physiology for Nursing and Healthcare Students at a Glance, Second Edition. Ian Peate.
© 2022 John Wiley & Sons Ltd. Published 2022 by John Wiley & Sons Ltd.
Companion website: www.wiley.com/go/peate/anatomyandphysiology

The liver

The liver is the largest solid organ in the body. In the adult, the liver can weigh up to 1.5 kilograms. It is situated in the upper right aspect of the abdomen, just under the rib cage and below the diaphragm (the muscle below the lungs and heart that separates the chest cavity from the abdomen).

Two major types of cells populate the liver lobes: parenchymal and non-parenchymal cells; 80% of the liver volume is occupied by parenchymal cells, commonly referred to as hepatocytes. Non-parenchymal cells constitute 40% of the total number of liver cells but only 6.5% of its volume.

Segments of the liver

The liver is divided into segments (Figure 29.1). Each segment of the liver is further divided into lobules (Figure 29.2). Lobules are usually represented as discrete hexagonal clusters of hepatocytes. The hepatocytes assemble as plates which radiate from a central vein. Lobules are served by arterial, venous and biliary vessels at their periphery. Liver lobules have little connective tissue separating one lobule from another. The paucity of connective tissue makes it more difficult to identify the portal triads and the boundaries of individual lobules. Central veins are easier to identify due to their large lumen and because they lack connective tissue that provides the portal triad vessels.

Ligaments of the liver

The coronary ligament attaches the liver (from the diaphragmatic surface) to the diaphragm. It is an irregular fold of peritoneum and surrounds the triangular base of the diaphragmatic surface. It is continuous with the outermost layer of the caudal vena cava. The falciform ligament is ventral to the coronary ligament. It is located cranial to the umbilicus and is a remnant of the umbilical vein. The triangular ligament is on the right and left sides of the coronary ligament.

Blood supply

The liver receives a dual blood supply from the hepatic portal vein and the hepatic arteries. The hepatic portal vein supplies 75% of the blood supply. This venous blood is drained from the spleen, gastrointestinal tract and other organs. The hepatic arteries supply arterial blood to the liver, accounting for the remainder of its blood flow. Oxygen is provided from both vessels; approximately half of the liver's oxygen demand is met by the hepatic portal vein and half by the hepatic arteries.

The hepatic artery comes off the coeliac trunk which in turn comes from the aorta. The venous blood from the digestive tract is collected by the portal vein, which then supplies blood to the liver. The hepatic veins drain blood from the liver into the inferior vena cava. Branches of the hepatic artery and vein and the bile duct flow into the liver. Collectively, these three vessels are termed the portal triad and they are located at the corners of the liver lobules (see Figure 29.2).

Functions of the liver

Nearly all the blood circulated around the abdomen flows back through the portal vein to the liver where it comes in contact with the liver cells, ensuring the products of digestion are brought to the hepatic cells before entering the general circulation. Other functions include production of bile, carbohydrate metabolism, glycogenesis, glycogenolysis, gluconeogenesis and the breakdown of insulin and other hormones. Protein metabolism produces soluble mediators of the clotting cascade, albumin and hormone-transporting globulins. The liver is also involved in lipid metabolism, lipogenesis and the synthesis of cholesterol.

It also has a role in immunoregulation via the Kupffer cells and complement synthesis and metabolism. The liver is important in storage of water-soluble and fat-soluble vitamins, iron, triglyceride and glycogen.

The liver breaks down haemoglobin and toxic substances through drug metabolism. It converts ammonia to urea and regulates the management of waste of metabolism, such as haem and ammonia (amino acids).

The gall bladder

The gall bladder is a small green muscular sac that lies posterior to the liver. It functions as a reservoir for bile until it is required for digestion. It also concentrates bile by absorbing water. The mucosa of the gall bladder, like the rugae of the stomach, contains folds that allow the gall bladder to stretch in order to accommodate varying volumes of bile. When the smooth muscle walls of the gall bladder contract, bile is expelled into the cystic duct and down into the common bile duct before entering the duodenum via the hepatopancreatic ampulla.

The function of bile

When food containing fat enters the digestive tract, it stimulates the secretion of cholecystokinin (CCK) (a hormone). In response to CCK, the adult human gall bladder, which stores approximately 50 mL of bile, releases the bile into the duodenum. The bile emulsifies fats in partly digested food. During storage in the gall bladder, bile becomes more concentrated which increases its potency and intensifies its effect on fats (Figure 29.3).

Biliary tract

The biliary tract (or biliary tree) is the term for the path by which bile is secreted by the liver then transported to the first part of the small intestine, the duodenum. It is referred to as a tree because it begins with many small branches which end in the common bile duct, sometimes referred to as the trunk of the biliary tree (see Figure 29.3).

Clinical practice point

Hepatitis is inflammation of the liver, frequently the result of a viral infection or liver damage caused by drinking alcohol. There are several types of hepatitis. Some types of hepatitis will pass without any serious problems, others can be chronic in nature and cause scarring of the liver (cirrhosis), loss of liver function and, in some cases, liver cancer. Acute hepatitis often has no noticeable symptoms and the person may not realise that they have it. If symptoms develop, they can include myalgia, arthralgia, pyrexia, nausea and vomiting, malaise, anorexia, abdominal pain, dark urine and pale faeces, pruritus and jaundice. Chronic hepatitis may not have any obvious symptoms until liver failure occurs and it may only be diagnosed during blood tests. In the later stages, it can cause jaundice, leg and ankle oedema, confusion and blood in the faeces.

The pancreas and spleen

Figure 30.1 The pancreas.

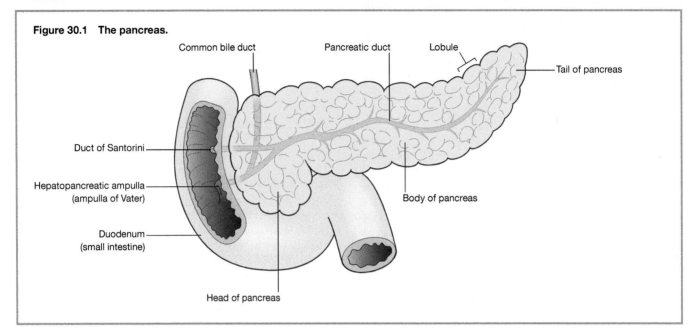

Anatomy and Physiology for Nursing and Healthcare Students at a Glance, Second Edition. Ian Peate.
© 2022 John Wiley & Sons Ltd. Published 2022 by John Wiley & Sons Ltd.
Companion website: www.wiley.com/go/peate/anatomyandphysiology

The pancreas

The pancreas is an abdominal glandular organ that has both digestive (exocrine) and hormonal (endocrine) functions. It lies close to a number of major vessels and significant landmarks in vascular **anatomy**. The aorta and inferior vena cava pass posterior to the head of the **pancreas.** The pancreas is approximately 12–15 cm long and 2.5 cm thick. It is situated across the back of the abdomen, behind the stomach. The head of the pancreas is on the right side of the abdomen and is connected to the duodenum (the first section of the small intestine) through a small tube called the pancreatic duct. The narrow end of the pancreas, called the tail, extends to the left side of the body (Figure 30.1).

The pancreatic juices are secreted by exocrine cells into small ducts that unite to form larger ducts. The duct of Wirsung is the larger of the two ducts and in most people this duct joins the common bile duct and enters the duodenum as a dilated common duct called the hepatopancreatic ampulla. In most people, there is a second smaller (minor or accessory) papilla, situated about 2 cm above the main papilla and slightly to its right. This is the exit place for Santorini's duct. The minor papilla occasionally takes over when the main papilla is not able to function correctly and becomes the main site of drainage for pancreatic juices.

The cells of the pancreas are responsible for making endocrine and exocrine products. The cells of the islets of Langerhans produce the endocrine hormones insulin and glucagon which control carbohydrate metabolism.

The composition of pancreatic juice

Two hormones regulate the secretion of pancreatic juice. Secretin is produced in response to the presence of hydrochloric acid in the duodenum that promotes the secretion of bicarbonate ions. Cholecystokinin, secreted in response to the intake of protein and fat, promotes secretion of the enzymes present in pancreatic juice. Parasympathetic vagus nerve stimulation also promotes the release of pancreatic juice.

The acini glands of the exocrine pancreas produce 1.2–1.5 L of pancreatic juice daily. Pancreatic juice is a clear colourless fluid consisting of water, mineral salts, the enzymes amylase and lipase and the inactive enzyme precursors trypsinogen, chymotrypsinogen and procarboxypeptidase. Pancreatic juice travels from the pancreas via the pancreatic duct into the duodenum at the hepatopancreatic ampulla.

The cells of the pancreatic ducts secrete bicarbonate ions which make pancreatic juice slightly alkaline pH (pH 7.1–8.2). This helps to neutralise acidic chyme from the stomach, thus protecting the small intestine from damage by the acidity, and stops the action of pepsin from the stomach. This provides a proper pH environment for the action of enzymes in the small intestine.

The functions of pancreatic juice

Functions include digestion of proteins: enteropeptidase converts trypsinogen and chymotrypsinogen into the active proteolytic enzymes trypsin and chymotrypsin. These activated enzymes convert polypeptides to tripeptides, dipeptides and amino acids. It also plays a role in digestion of carbohydrates; pancreatic amylase helps in the conversion of digestible polysaccharides (starch) not acted upon by salivary amylase to disaccharides. Bile salts help lipase in the conversion of fats to fatty acids and glycerol, by reducing the size of the globules resulting in an increased surface area.

The spleen

The spleen is an organ shaped like a shoe that lies relative to the 9th and 11th ribs and is located in the upper left quadrant and partly in the epigastrium. Thus, the spleen is situated between the fundus of the stomach and the diaphragm. The spleen is very vascular and reddish purple in colour; its size and weight vary.

The spleen is a soft organ that has a thin outer covering of tough connective tissue, known as a capsule.

The spleen contains two main types of tissue – white pulp and red pulp. White pulp is lymphatic tissue (material which is part of the immune system), mainly made up of white blood cells. Red pulp is made up of venous sinuses (blood-filled cavities) and splenic cords. Splenic cords are special tissues which contain different types of red and white blood cells.

The spleen has two coats: an external serous and an internal fibroelastic coat. The external or serous coat (tunica serosa) is derived from the peritoneum; it is thin, smooth and closely adherent to the fibroelastic coat.

The spleen receives blood through the splenic artery and blood leaves the spleen through the splenic vein. Although the spleen is connected to the blood vessels of the stomach and pancreas, it is not involved in digestion. Anything that relates to the spleen is referred to as splenic.

Functions of the spleen

Blood flows into the spleen where it enters the white pulp. Here, white blood cells called B and T cells screen the blood flowing through. T cells help to recognise invading pathogens (for example, bacteria and viruses) that might cause illness and then attack them. B cells make antibodies that help to stop infections from occurring.

Blood also enters red pulp. Red pulp has three main functions.

- It removes old and damaged red blood cells. Red blood cells have a lifespan of about 120 days. After this time they stop carrying oxygen effectively. Special cells called macrophages break down these old red blood cells. Haemoglobin found within the cells is also broken down and then recycled.
- Red pulp also stores up to one-third of the body's supply of platelets. Platelets are fragments of cells that circulate in the bloodstream, helping to stop bleeding when the blood vessel is cut. These extra stored platelets can be released from the spleen if severe bleeding occurs.
- In the foetus, red pulp can also aid in the production of new red blood cells.

The spleen is not essential to life. Other organs such as the liver and bone marrow are able to take over many of its functions.

Clinical practice point

Acute pancreatitis is a condition in which the pancreas becomes inflamed over a short period of time. Most people with acute pancreatitis will start to feel better within about a week and have no further problems. However, some people with severe acute pancreatitis can go on to develop serious complications. The most common symptoms of acute pancreatitis include sudden-onset severe pain in the centre of the abdomen, feeling nauseous and vomiting, diarrhoea and pyrexia. Acute pancreatitis is very often associated with gall stones or drinking too much alcohol, but sometimes the cause is not known. The overall aim of treatment for acute pancreatitis is to help control the condition and manage any symptoms. Admission to hospital is usually required. Intravenous fluids are required, pain relief is given and oxygen prescribed. Treatment is provided in response to individual needs.

31 Digestion

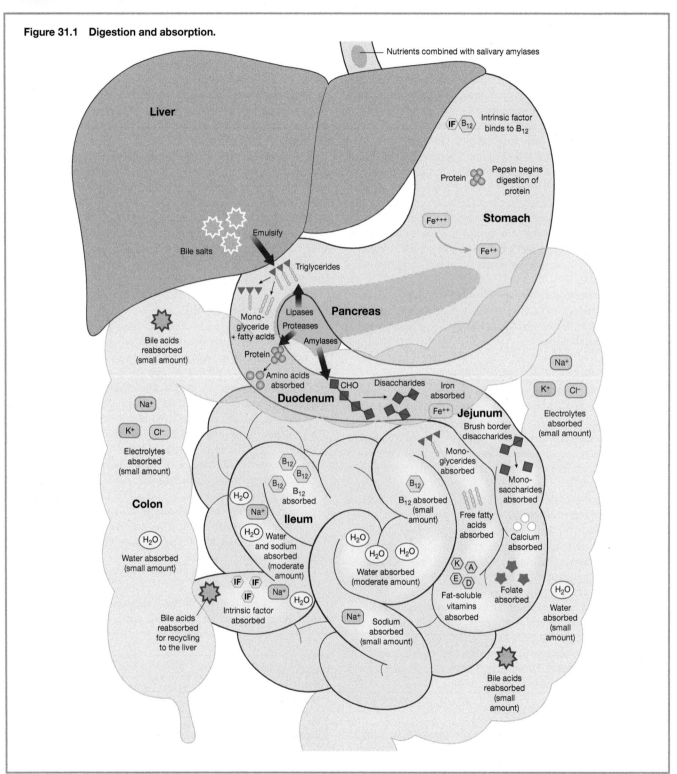

Figure 31.1   Digestion and absorption.

Anatomy and Physiology for Nursing and Healthcare Students at a Glance, Second Edition. Ian Peate.
© 2022 John Wiley & Sons Ltd. Published 2022 by John Wiley & Sons Ltd.
Companion website: www.wiley.com/go/peate/anatomyandphysiology

Digestion is a form of catabolism – the breakdown of macro food molecules to smaller ones (Figure 31.1).

Mechanical digestion

Mechanical digestion is simply the aspect of digestion that is achieved through a mechanism or movement.

Mastication

The first step in digestion begins as soon as the food enters the mouth. Mastication (chewing) begins the process of breaking down food into nutrients.

Peristalsis

Mechanical digestion also involves the process known as peristalsis. Peristalsis is the involuntary contractions that are responsible for the movement of food through the oesophagus and intestinal tract.

In the stomach, there are three layers of muscle, longitudinal, circular and oblique, which together contract and relax to form the churning motion which mixes the food. This mixing aids in digestion as it begins to break up the food and also increases the contact the food has with enzymes and acids in the gastric juice. Bile salts also act to emulsify large fat globules into smaller fat droplets.

Chemical digestion

Chemical digestion is achieved with the addition of chemicals to the food. Digestive enzymes and water are responsible for the breakdown of complex molecules such as fats, proteins and carbohydrates into smaller molecules. These smaller molecules can then be absorbed for use by cells.

The presence of these digestive enzymes accelerates the digestion process, whereas the absence of these enzymes slows overall reaction speed. Digestive enzymes mainly responsible for chemical digestion include the following.

Protease

Any of various enzymes, including the proteinases and peptidases that catalyse the hydrolytic breakdown of proteins. Proteolytic enzymes are very important in digestion as they break the peptide bonds in the protein foods to liberate the amino acids that are needed by the body.

Collagenase

Enzymes that break the peptide bonds in collagen. Collagens are the major fibrous component of extracellular connective tissue.

Lipase

Lipids are one of the three major food groups needed for good nutrition. Lipase is the digestive enzyme needed to digest fat. It hydrolyses lipids, the ester bonds in triglycerides, to form fatty acids and glycerol.

Fats require special digestive action before absorption because the end products must be carried in a water medium (blood and lymph) in which fats are not soluble. Lipase is the primary enzyme used to split fats into fatty acids and glycerol. Although little actual fat digestion occurs in the stomach, gastric lipase does digest already emulsified fats such as in egg yolk and cream.

Amylase

Any of a group of enzymes that catalyse the hydrolysis of starch to sugar to produce carbohydrate derivatives. Amylase is present in saliva, where it begins the process of digestion. Foods that contain much starch but little sugar, such as rice and potato, taste slightly sweet as they are chewed because amylase turns some of their starch into sugar in the mouth. The pancreas also makes amylase (alpha-amylase) to hydrolyse dietary starch into disaccharides and trisaccharides which are converted by other enzymes to glucose to supply the body with energy.

Trypsin

A proteolytic digestive enzyme produced by the exocrine pancreas. It speeds up the chemical reaction, in the small intestine of the breakdown of dietary proteins to peptones, peptides and amino acids. When the pancreas is stimulated by cholecystokinin, it is then secreted into the first part of the small intestine (the duodenum) via the pancreatic duct. Once in the small intestine, the enzyme enteropeptidase activates it into trypsin.

Chymotrypsin

A proteolytic enzyme produced by the pancreas that catalyses the hydrolysis of casein and gelatin. Chymotrypsin is a serine endopeptidase produced by the acinar cells of the pancreas.

Digestion and absorption

Carbohydrate

Monosaccharides, such as glucose, galactose and fructose, are produced by the breakdown of polysaccharides and are transported to the intestinal epithelium by facilitated diffusion or active transport. Facilitated diffusion moves the sugars into the bloodstream.

Protein

Proteins are broken down to peptide fragments by pepsin in the stomach and by pancreatic trypsin and chymotrypsin in the small intestine. The fragments are then digested to free amino acids by carboxypeptidase from the pancreas and aminopeptidase from the intestinal epithelium. Free amino acids enter the epithelium by secondary active transport and leave it by facilitated diffusion. Small amounts of intact proteins can enter interstitial fluid by endo- and exocytosis.

Fat

Fat digestion occurs by pancreatic lipase in the small intestine. Large lipid droplets are first broken down into smaller droplets by a process called emulsification. Pancreatic colipase binds the water-soluble lipase to the lipid substrate.

Vitamins

Fat-soluble vitamins are absorbed and stored along with fats. Most water-soluble vitamins are absorbed by diffusion or mediated transport. Vitamin B12, because of its large size and charged nature, first binds to a protein, called intrinsic factor, which is secreted by the stomach epithelium and is then absorbed by endocytosis.

Water

Most of the material absorbed from the cavity of the small intestine is water in which salt is dissolved. The salt and water come from the food and liquid that is swallowed and the juices secreted by the many digestive glands.

> **Clinical practice point**
> Gastro-oesophageal reflux disease (GORD) (heartburn) is a common condition, where acid from the stomach leaks up into the oesophagus. It can occur due to weakening of the ring of muscle at the bottom of the oesophagus. GORD causes symptoms such as heartburn and an unpleasant taste in the back of the mouth. It may be an occasional nuisance for some people but for others it can be a severe, lifelong problem. GORD can often be controlled with self-help measures and medication. Occasionally, surgery may be needed to correct the problem.

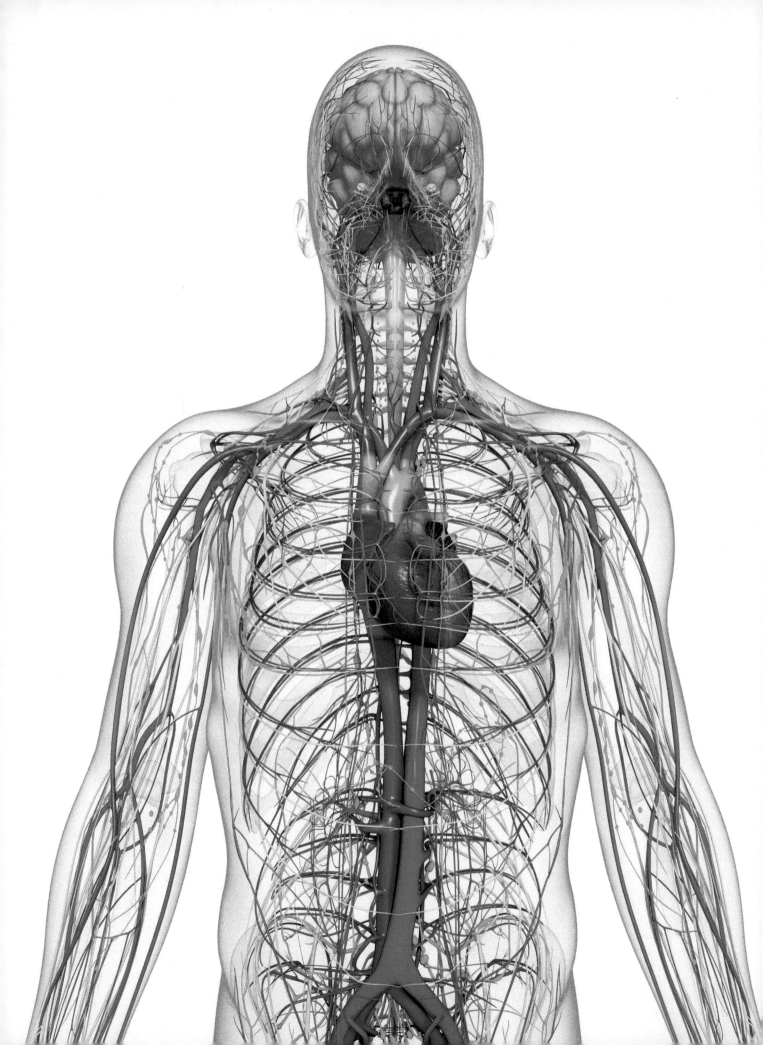

The urinary system

Part 6

Chapters

32 The kidney (microscopic)

Figure 32.1   A nephron.

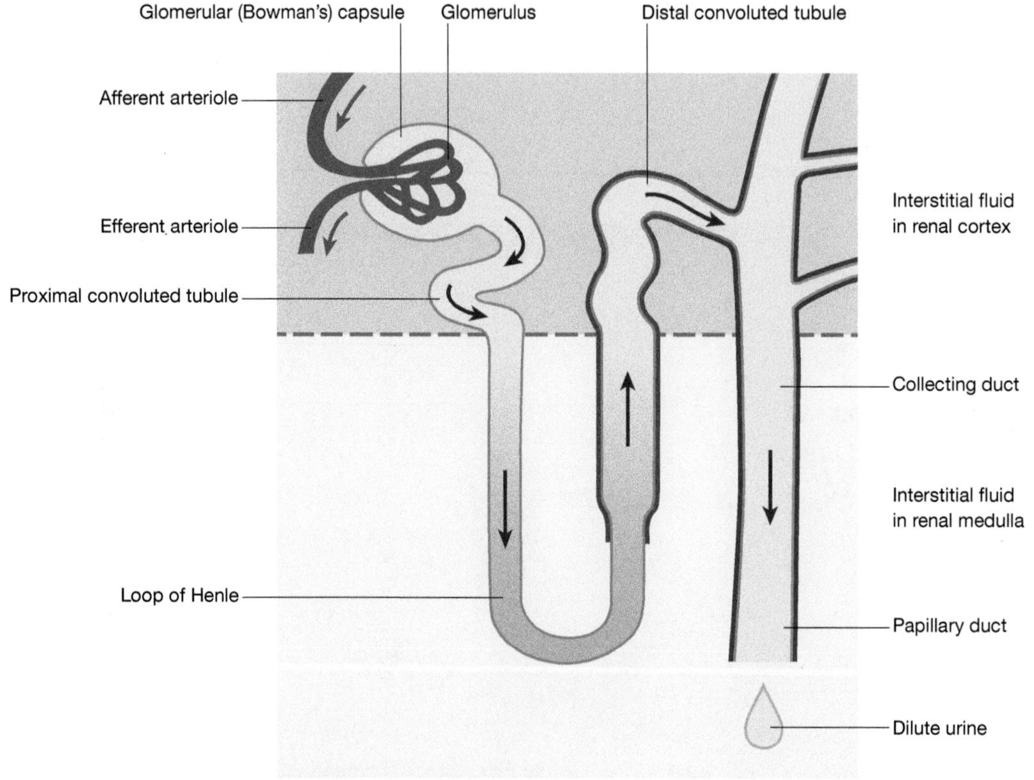

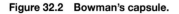

Glomerular (Bowman's) capsule   Glomerulus   Distal convoluted tubule

Afferent arteriole

Efferent arteriole

Proximal convoluted tubule

Interstitial fluid in renal cortex

Collecting duct

Interstitial fluid in renal medulla

Loop of Henle

Papillary duct

Dilute urine

Source: Peate I & Nair M. Fundamentals of Anatomy and Physiology for Student Nurses (2011).

Figure 32.2   Bowman's capsule.

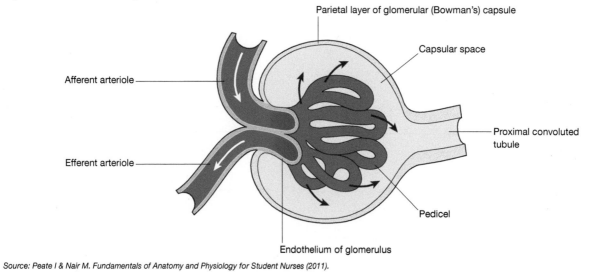

Parietal layer of glomerular (Bowman's) capsule

Capsular space

Afferent arteriole

Proximal convoluted tubule

Efferent arteriole

Pedicel

Endothelium of glomerulus

Source: Peate I & Nair M. Fundamentals of Anatomy and Physiology for Student Nurses (2011).

Anatomy and Physiology for Nursing and Healthcare Students at a Glance, Second Edition. Ian Peate.
© 2022 John Wiley & Sons Ltd. Published 2022 by John Wiley & Sons Ltd.
Companion website: www.wiley.com/go/peate/anatomyandphysiology

Nephrons

The nephrons are small structures which form the functional units of the kidney. The nephron consists of a glomerulus and a renal tubule (Figure 32.1). The renal tubule can be further divided into Bowman's capsule, proximal convoluted tubule, loop of Henle, distal convoluted tubule and collecting ducts. There are over 1 million nephrons in each kidney and it is in these structures that urine is formed. The key function of the nephron is to regulate water and electrolytes by filtering the blood, reabsorbing what is needed and excreting the rest as urine. A nephron eliminates waste from the body, regulates blood volume and blood pressure, controls levels of electrolytes and metabolites and regulates blood pH.

Bowman's capsule

Also known as a glomerular capsule, this is a cup-like sac and is the first portion of the nephron. A Bowman's capsule is part of the filtration system in the kidneys (Figure 32.2). When blood reaches the kidneys for filtration, it enters the Bowman's capsule first, with the capsule separating the blood into two components: a filtrated blood product and a filtrate which is moved through the nephron. The Bowman's capsule consists of visceral and parietal layers. The visceral layer is lined by epithelial cells called podocytes while the parietal layer is lined with simple squamous epithelium, and it is in the Bowman's capsule that the network of capillaries called the glomerulus is found.

Glomerulus

The glomerulus consists of a tight network of capillaries surrounded by podocytes. Podocytes have narrow cell processes that in turn give rise to secondary extensions called pedicels (see Figure 32.2). Podocytes completely surround the capillary network. As blood flows through the glomerulus, water and metabolic waste are filtered through the capillary walls by the surrounding podocytes. Water and waste pass into the Bowman's capsule.

Proximal convoluted tubule

From the Bowman's capsule, the filtrate drains into the proximal convoluted tubule (see Figure 32.1). The surface of the epithelial cells of this segment of the nephron is covered with densely packed microvilli which increase the surface area of the cells, thus facilitating their resorptive function. The in-folded membranes forming the microvilli are the site of numerous sodium pumps. Reabsorption of salt, water and glucose from the glomerular filtrate occurs in this section of the tubule; at the same time certain substances, including uric acid and drug metabolites, are actively transferred from the blood capillaries into the tubule for excretion.

Loop of Henle

In the kidney, the loop of Henle is the portion of a nephron that leads from the proximal convoluted tubule to the distal convoluted tubule. It can be divided into two sections: the descending and ascending loops (see Figure 32.1). The thin descending limb has low permeability to ions and urea, while being highly permeable to water. The loop has a sharp bend in the renal medulla going from the descending to the ascending thin limb.

The thin ascending loop is impermeable to water but is permeable to ions. Sodium (Na^+), potassium (K^+) and chloride (Cl^-) ions are reabsorbed from the urine by secondary active transport by a Na-K-Cl co-transporter. The electrical and concentration gradient drives more reabsorption of Na^+, as well as other cations such as magnesium (Mg^{2+}) and calcium (Ca^{2+}).

The loop of Henle is supplied by blood in a series of straight capillaries descending from the cortical efferent arterioles. These capillaries (vasa recta) also have a countercurrent multiplier mechanism that prevents washout of solutes from the medulla, thereby maintaining the medullary concentration. As water is osmotically moved from the descending limb into the interstitium, it readily enters the vasa recta. The low blood flow through the vasa recta allows time for osmotic equilibration and can be altered by changing the resistance of the vessels' efferent arterioles.

Distal convoluted tubule

The distal convoluted tubule is a twisted, tube-like structure of the nephron (see Figure 32.1). It is the section farthest away from the renal corpuscle, and the cells that line it are able to actively pump potentially harmful substances, such as ammonia, urea and certain drugs, out of the blood and into the urine. From the distal convoluted tubule, useful substances are returned to the blood, while waste products and toxins are added to the filtrate. Hydrogen ions are also pumped in, making the urine pH more acidic. The distal convoluted tubule walls do not normally allow water to pass through, but the hormone ADH can open channels which allow water to move out, concentrating the urine.

Collecting ducts

From the distal convoluted tubule, filtrate drains into what are known as collecting ducts (see Figure 32.1). These are tubes which receive filtrate from the distal convoluted tubules of many nephrons. Inside these collecting ducts, water can be absorbed to regulate the final concentration of urine produced by the kidneys. On leaving the collecting ducts, urine enters a space known as the renal pelvis, from where it passes into the bladder and is expelled from the body during urination.

The collecting duct system is under the control of ADH. In the absence of ADH, water in the renal filtrate is allowed to enter the urine, promoting diuresis. When ADH is present, aquaporins aid reabsorption of water, thereby inhibiting diuresis.

Clinical practice point

Chronic kidney disease (CKD) is a long-term condition in which the kidneys do not work as well as they should. It is a common condition often associated with getting older. It can affect anyone but is more common in people who are black or of south Asian origin. Over time, CKD can get worse and eventually the kidneys may cease working altogether, although this is uncommon. Many people with CKD are able to live long lives with the condition. Often, in the early stages there are no symptoms. It may only be diagnosed if the person has had a blood or urine test for another reason. At a more advanced stage, symptoms can include fatigue, oedematous legs, feet and hands, shortness of breath, nausea and haematuria. CKD is usually caused by other conditions that put a strain on the kidneys. Often it is the result of a combination of different problems. CKD can be caused by hypertension, diabetes mellitus, hypercholesterolaemia, kidney infections, glomerulonephritis, polycystic kidney disease, outflow obstruction (such as kidney stones, prostatic enlargement) and long-term, regular use of some medicines, for example lithium and non-steroidal anti-inflammatory drugs.

33 The kidney (macroscopic)

Figure 33.1 External layers of the kidney.

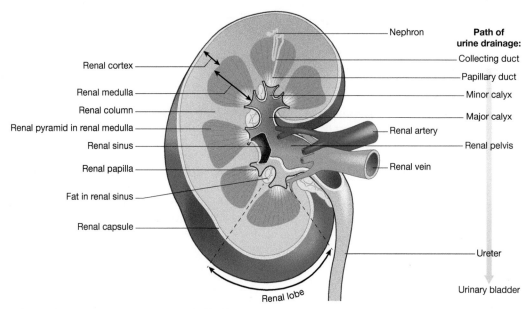

Source: Peate I, Wild K & Nair M (eds). Nursing Practice: Knowledge and Care (2014).

Figure 33.2 Blood flow through the kidney.

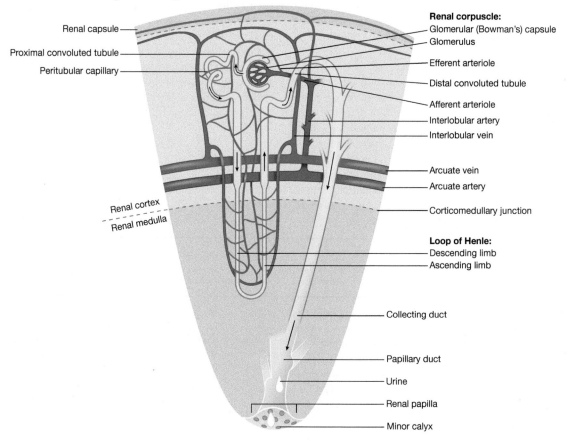

Anatomy and Physiology for Nursing and Healthcare Students at a Glance, Second Edition. Ian Peate.
© 2022 John Wiley & Sons Ltd. Published 2022 by John Wiley & Sons Ltd.
Companion website: www.wiley.com/go/peate/anatomyandphysiology

The kidney

There are usually two kidneys, one on each side of the spinal column (located in the posterior abdomen, retroperitoneally). They are approximately 11 cm long, 5–6 cm wide and 3–4 cm thick. The adrenal glands sit immediately superior to the kidneys. They are bean-shaped organs where the outer border is convex; the inner border is known as the hilum (or hilus) and it is here that the renal arteries, renal veins, nerves and ureters enter and leave the kidneys (Figure 33.1). The renal artery carries blood to the kidneys and once the blood is filtered, the renal vein takes the blood away. The right kidney is in contact with the liver's large right lobe and hence the right kidney is approximately 2–4 cm lower than the left kidney.

Each kidney is covered by three layers: the renal fascia, adipose tissue and renal capsule. The renal fascia is the outer layer and consists of a thin layer of connective tissue that anchors the kidneys to the abdominal wall and the surrounding tissues. The middle layer is called the adipose tissue which surrounds the capsule. It cushions the kidneys from trauma. The inner layer is the renal capsule which consists of a layer of smooth connective tissue that is continuous with the outer layer of the ureter. The renal capsule protects the kidneys from trauma and maintains their shape.

The main function of the kidneys is to filter and excrete waste products from the blood. They also have a responsibility for water and electrolyte balance in the body.

Renal cortex

The renal cortex is the outer portion of the kidney between the renal capsule and renal medulla. In the adult, it forms a continuous smooth outer zone with a number of projections (cortical columns) that extend down between the pyramids. It contains the renal corpuscles and the renal tubules except for parts of the loop of Henle which descend into the renal medulla. It also contains blood vessels and cortical collecting ducts.

Renal medulla

The renal medulla is the innermost portion of the kidney. The medulla is lighter in colour and it has an abundance of blood vessels and tubules of the nephron. The renal medulla (pyramid) is composed of conical masses of tissue called renal pyramids, whose bases are directed toward the convex surface of the kidney, and whose apices form the renal papillae. The renal cortex forms a shell around the medulla. Its tissues dip into the medulla between adjacent renal pyramids to form renal columns. The granular appearance of the cortex is due to the random arrangement of tiny tubules associated with nephrons, the functional units of the kidney.

Renal pelvis

The renal pelvis forms the expanded upper portion of the ureter, which is funnel shaped, and is the region where two or three calyces converge. These are cavities in which urine collects before it flows on into the urinary bladder. The renal pelvis is lined with a moist mucous membrane layer that is only a few cells thick; the membrane is attached to a thicker coating of smooth muscle fibres which in turn is surrounded by a layer of connective tissue. The mucous membrane of the pelvis is somewhat folded so that there is some room for tissue expansion when urine distends the pelvis.

The muscle fibres are arranged in longitudinal and circular layers. Contractions of the muscle layers occur in periodic waves known as peristaltic movements. The peristaltic waves help to push the urine from the pelvis into the ureter and bladder. The lining of the pelvis and the ureter is impermeable to the normal substances found in urine; thus, the walls of these structures do not absorb fluids.

Blood supply

The renal artery enters into the kidney at the level of the first lumbar vertebra, just below the superior mesenteric artery. The renal circulation receives approximately 20–25% of the cardiac output. It branches from the abdominal aorta and returns blood to the ascending vena cava. Each renal artery branches into segmental arteries, dividing further into interlobar arteries which penetrate the renal capsule and extend through the renal columns between the renal pyramids. The interlobar arteries then supply blood to the arcuate arteries that run through the boundary of the cortex and medulla. Each arcuate artery supplies several interlobular arteries feeding into the afferent arterioles that supply the glomeruli (Figure 33.2).

From here, efferent arterioles leave the glomerulus and divide into peritubular capillaries. These drain into the interlobular veins and then into the arcuate vein and then into the interlobar vein, which runs into the lobar vein, which opens into the segmental vein, which drains into the renal vein, and then blood moves into the inferior vena cava.

Nerve supply

The kidney and nervous system communicate via the renal plexus, whose fibres course along the renal arteries to reach each kidney. Input from the sympathetic nervous system triggers vasoconstriction in the kidney, thereby reducing renal blood flow. The kidney also receives input from the parasympathetic nervous system, by way of the renal branches of the vagus nerve (cranial nerve X). Sensory input from the kidney travels to the T10–11 levels of the spinal cord and is sensed in the corresponding dermatome.

Clinical practice point

Dialysis removes waste products and excess fluid from the blood when the kidneys no longer function effectively. If the kidneys are malfunctioning, for example if the patient has chronic kidney disease (kidney failure), the kidneys may no longer be able to filter the blood appropriately. As a result of this, waste products and fluid can build up to dangerous levels in the body. If this is left untreated, it could cause a number of unwanted symptoms and may eventually be fatal. Dialysis filters out unwanted substances and fluids from the blood before this happens. In some cases, kidney failure may be a temporary problem and dialysis can be stopped when the kidneys recover. Often someone with kidney failure will require a kidney transplant. It is not always possible to carry out a kidney transplant immediately, so dialysis could be needed until a suitable donor kidney becomes available. If a kidney transplant is not appropriate, dialysis may be required for the rest of the person's life.

34 The ureters, bladder and urethra

Figure 34.1   Blood supply to the ureter.

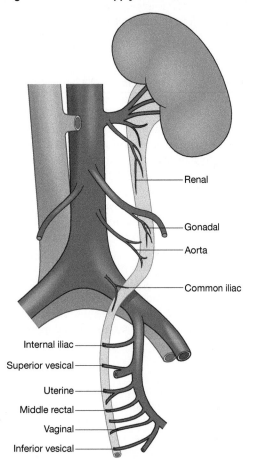

- Renal
- Gonadal
- Aorta
- Common iliac
- Internal iliac
- Superior vesical
- Uterine
- Middle rectal
- Vaginal
- Inferior vesical

Figure 34.3   The male urethra.

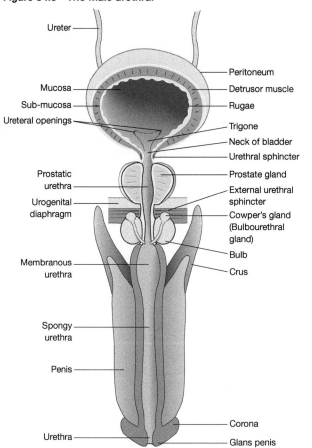

- Ureter
- Mucosa
- Sub-mucosa
- Ureteral openings
- Peritoneum
- Detrusor muscle
- Rugae
- Trigone
- Neck of bladder
- Urethral sphincter
- Prostatic urethra
- Urogenital diaphragm
- Prostate gland
- External urethral sphincter
- Cowper's gland (Bulbourethral gland)
- Membranous urethra
- Bulb
- Crus
- Spongy urethra
- Penis
- Corona
- Urethra
- Glans penis

Source: Peate I & Nair M. Fundamentals of Anatomy and Physiology for Student Nurses (2011).

Figure 34.2   The urinary bladder.

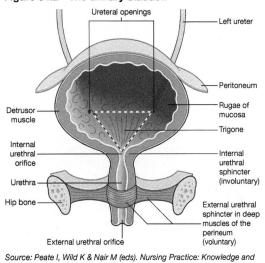

- Ureteral openings
- Left ureter
- Peritoneum
- Detrusor muscle
- Rugae of mucosa
- Trigone
- Internal urethral orifice
- Internal urethral sphincter (involuntary)
- Urethra
- Hip bone
- External urethral sphincter in deep muscles of the perineum (voluntary)
- External urethral orifice

Source: Peate I, Wild K & Nair M (eds). Nursing Practice: Knowledge and Care (2014).

Figure 34.4   The female urethra.

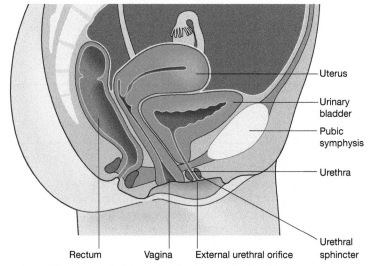

- Uterus
- Urinary bladder
- Pubic symphysis
- Urethra
- Urethral sphincter
- Rectum
- Vagina
- External urethral orifice

Source: Peate I, Wild K & Nair M (eds). Nursing Practice: Knowledge and Care (2014).

Anatomy and Physiology for Nursing and Healthcare Students at a Glance, Second Edition. Ian Peate.
© 2022 John Wiley & Sons Ltd. Published 2022 by John Wiley & Sons Ltd.
Companion website: www.wiley.com/go/peate/anatomyandphysiology

The ureters

The ureters transport urine from the pelvis of the kidney to the bladder. The flow of urine occurs via peristaltic contraction of the muscular walls of the ureter. Approximately 1–5 peristaltic waves form every minute, depending on the formation of urine.

The abdominal ureter

The ureter is roughly 25–30 cm long in adults and courses down the retroperitoneum in an 'S' curve. At the proximal end of the ureter is the renal pelvis; at the distal end is the bladder. The ureter begins at the level of the renal artery and vein posterior to these structures.

The pelvic ureter

The ureter enters the pelvis, where it crosses anteriorly to the iliac vessels, which usually occurs at the bifurcation of the common iliac artery into the internal and external iliac arteries. Here, the ureters are within 5 cm of one another before they diverge laterally.

Blood supply

The vascular supply and venous drainage of the ureter are derived from varied and numerous vessels. In the abdominal ureter, the arterial supply is located on the medial aspect of the ureter, whereas in the pelvic ureter, the lateral aspect is the area for the blood supply (Figure 34.1).

The urinary bladder

The urinary bladder is a hollow muscular organ which stores urine, located in the pelvic cavity posterior to the symphysis pubis. In the male, the bladder lies anterior to the rectum and in the female it lies anterior to the vagina and inferior to the uterus. When the bladder is empty, the inner section forms folds (rugae) but as the bladder fills up with urine, the walls of the bladder become smoother (Figure 34.2). The bladder normally distends and holds approximately 300–350 mL of urine. In females, the bladder is slightly smaller because the uterus occupies the space above the bladder.

Layers of the bladder

The bladder is composed of three layers. The serous coat (tunica serosa) is a partial one and is derived from the peritoneum. The muscular coat (tunica muscularis) consists of three layers of unstripped muscular fibres: an external layer composed of fibres having for the most part a longitudinal arrangement; a middle layer, in which the fibres are arranged, more or less, in a circular manner; and an internal layer, in which the fibres have a general longitudinal arrangement. The mucous coat (tunica mucosa) is thin, smooth and of a pale rose colour. It is continuous through the ureters with the lining membrane of the renal tubules and below with that of the urethra.

Vessels and nerves

The bladder is supplied by the superior, middle and inferior vesical arteries, derived from the anterior trunk of the hypogastric artery. The obturator and inferior gluteal arteries also supply small visceral branches to the bladder and in the female additional branches are derived from the uterine and vaginal arteries.

The nerves of the bladder are (i) fine medullated fibres from the third and fourth sacral nerves, and (ii) non-medullated fibres from the hypogastric plexus.

The urethra

The urethra is a muscular tube that drains urine from the bladder and conveys it out of the body. It contains three coats –muscular, erectile and mucous. The muscular coat is the continuation of the bladder muscle layer. The urethra is encompassed by two separate urethral sphincter muscles. The internal urethral sphincter is formed by involuntary smooth muscles while the lower voluntary muscles make up the external sphincter. The internal sphincter is created by the detrusor muscle. Sphincters keep the urethra closed when urine is not being passed. The internal urethral sphincter is under involuntary control and lies at the bladder–urethral junction. The external urethral sphincter is under voluntary control.

The male urethra

In the male, the urethra not only excretes urine but is also part of the reproductive system. Rather than the straight tube found in the female body, the male urethra is shaped like a 'S' to follow the line of the penis. It is approximately 20 cm long (Figure 34.3). The male urethra passes through three regions: the prostatic, membranous (shortest and least distensible portion of the urethra) and penile urethra (the region that spans the corpus spongiosum of the penis).

The prostatic portion is only about 2.5 cm long and passes along the neck of the urinary bladder through the prostate gland. This section is designed to accept drainage from the tiny ducts within the prostate and is equipped with two ejaculatory tubes.

The female urethra

The female urethra is bound to the anterior vaginal wall. The external opening of the urethra is anterior to the vagina and posterior to the clitoris. In the female, the urethra is approximately 4 cm long and leads out of the body via the urethral orifice. The urethral orifice is located in the vestibule in the labia minora. This can be found located in between the clitoris and the vaginal orifice (Figure 34.4). In the female, the urethras only function is to transport urine out of the body.

Clinical practice point

Urinary incontinence is the unintentional passing of urine. It is a common problem that is thought to affect millions of people. There are several types of urinary incontinence including stress incontinence – when urine leaks out at times when the bladder is under pressure, for example when the person coughs or laughs; urge incontinence – when urine leaks as the person feels a sudden, intense urge to urinate, or soon afterwards; overflow incontinence (chronic urinary retention) – when the person is unable to fully empty the bladder, which results in frequent leaking; total incontinence – when the bladder cannot store any urine at all, causing the person to pass urine constantly or have frequent leaking. It is also possible to have a mixture of both stress and urge urinary incontinence.

35 The formation of urine

Figure 35.1 Renal filtration.

Parietal layer of glomerular (Bowman's) capsule

Capsular space

Afferent arteriole

Efferent arteriole

Proximal convoluted tubule

Pedicel

Endothelium of glomerulus

Figure 35.2 Renin-angiotensin pathway.

- Low Na⁺
- Low BP
- Low volume
- Beta-adrenoceptors stimulate juxtaglomerular cells to release renin

Inhibited by ACE inhibitors used in hypertension and heart failure

Inhibited by AT1 receptor antagonists used in hypertension and heart failure

Renin

ACE

AII

Angiotensinogen → Proteolytic activation → AI → Proteolytic activation → AII

Vasoconstriction: increase in blood pressure

Aldosterone: acts on the distal tubules in the kidney to cause Na⁺ (and H₂O) retention to increase volume

Source: Randall MD (ed). Medical Sciences at a Glance (2014).

Anatomy and Physiology for Nursing and Healthcare Students at a Glance, Second Edition. Ian Peate.
© 2022 John Wiley & Sons Ltd. Published 2022 by John Wiley & Sons Ltd.
Companion website: www.wiley.com/go/peate/anatomyandphysiology

There are three processes involved in the formation of urine: filtration, selective reabsorption and secretion.

Filtration

Urine formation begins with the process of filtration of the blood, which is a continuous activity. As the blood passes through the glomeruli, much of its fluid, containing both useful chemicals and dissolved waste materials, flows out of the blood through the membranes (by osmosis and diffusion) where it is filtered and then flows into the Bowman's capsule. This process is called glomerular filtration (Figure 35.1). The water, waste products, salt, glucose and other chemicals that have been filtered out of the blood are known collectively as glomerular filtrate. The glomerular filtrate consists primarily of water, excess salts (sodium and potassium), glucose and a waste product called urea. Urea is created in the body to eliminate the very toxic ammonia products formed in the liver from the amino acids. Since humans are unable to excrete ammonia, it has to be converted to the less dangerous urea and then it is filtered out of the blood. Urea is the most abundant of the waste products that must be excreted by the kidneys.

Selective reabsorption

The proximal convoluted tubule has a microvillous cell border which increases the surface area for absorption from filtrate. There are also a large number of mitochondria which produce the extra adenosine triphosphate (ATP) required for active transport. Substances reabsorbed back into the bloodstream are water, glucose and other nutrients, and sodium and other ions. Reabsorption begins in the proximal convoluted tubules and continues in the loop of Henle, distal convoluted tubules and collecting tubules. Only 1% of the glomerular filtrate actually leaves the body and the remaining 99% is reabsorbed back into the bloodstream.

Blood glucose is entirely reabsorbed back into the blood from the proximal tubules; it is actively transported out of the tubules and into the peritubular capillary blood. None of this valuable nutrient is wasted by being lost in the urine.

Other components, such as ammonia and urea, are secreted rather than absorbed, while there are certain ions, including potassium, that can be both secreted and absorbed by the tubules according to the overall ionic balance throughout the body.

Secretion

Any substances not removed through filtration are then secreted into the renal tubules from the peritubular capillaries of the nephron; these include drugs and hydrogen ions. Tubular secretion mainly takes place by active transport, a process by which substances are moved across the biological membrane. Tubular secretion occurs from epithelial cells that line the renal tubules and the collecting ducts.

Substances secreted are hydrogen ions, potassium ions, ammonia and certain drugs.

Kidney tubule secretion plays a crucial role in maintaining the body's acid–base balance, another example of an important body function in which the kidneys participate.

Hormonal control

There are four hormones that play a role in the regulation of fluid and electrolytes: antidiuretic hormone (ADH), angiotensin, aldosterone and atrial natriuretic peptide (ANP).

Antidiuretic hormone

ADH is produced by the hypothalamus gland and stored in the posterior pituitary gland. This hormone increases the permeability of the cells in the distal convoluted tubule and collecting ducts. In the presence of ADH, more water is reabsorbed from the renal tubules and therefore the person will pass less urine. In the absence of ADH, less water is reabsorbed and the individual will pass more urine. Thus ADH plays a major role in the regulation of fluid balance in the body.

Angiotensin

Renin-angiotensin is a hormone system that regulates blood pressure and water (fluid) balance. When blood volume is low, the juxtaglomerular cells in the kidneys secrete renin directly into circulation. Plasma renin then carries out the conversion of angiotensinogen released by the liver to angiotensin I. Angiotensin I is subsequently converted to angiotensin II by the angiotensin-converting enzyme found in the lungs. Angiotensin II is a potent vasoactive peptide that causes blood vessels to constrict, resulting in increased blood pressure. It also stimulates the secretion of the hormone aldosterone from the adrenal cortex. Aldosterone causes the tubules of the kidneys to increase the reabsorption of sodium and water into the blood. This increases the volume of fluid in the body, which also increases blood pressure (Figure 35.2).

Aldosterone

This is a steroid hormone secreted by the adrenal glands. Aldosterone serves as the principal regulator of the salt and water balance of the body and thus is categorised as a mineralocorticoid. It also has a small effect on the metabolism of fats, carbohydrates and proteins.

Several things will stimulate aldosterone secretion, for example, when potassium levels are too high, if there is less blood flow to the kidneys or if the blood pressure falls. The converse is that aldosterone secretion will decrease if potassium levels fall, blood flow in the kidneys increases, blood volume increases or if the person consumes too much salt.

Atrial natriuretic peptide

ANP is a peptide hormone secreted by myocytes of the cardiac atria, promoting salt and water excretion and lowering blood pressure. ANP acts to reduce the water, sodium and adipose loads on the circulatory system and by this means reduces blood pressure. ANP has exactly the opposite function to aldosterone that is secreted by the zona glomerulosa. Synthesis of ANP also takes place in the ventricles, brain, suprarenal glands and renal glands. It is released in response to atrial stretch.

Clinical practice point

While urinary tract infections (UTIs) are not generally serious, they should be diagnosed and treated quickly in order to reduce the risk of any complications. A UTI may be classed as either an upper UTI if it is in a kidney, or an infection of the ureters or a lower UTI if it is a cystitis (a bladder infection) or an infection of the urethra. It may be difficult to tell whether a child has a UTI; the symptoms can be vague and young children cannot easily communicate how they feel. General signs that could suggest that a child has a UTI include pyrexia, vomiting, lethargy, irritability, poor feeding, not gaining weight properly, while in very young children, there may be jaundice. More specific signs that could indicate that a child has a UTI include dysuria (pain or a burning sensation when urinating), frequency of micturition, the child may deliberately hold in their urine, a change in their normal toilet habits, for example, the child may wet themselves or wet the bed, abdominal pain, lower back pain, malodorous urine, haematuria and cloudy urine.

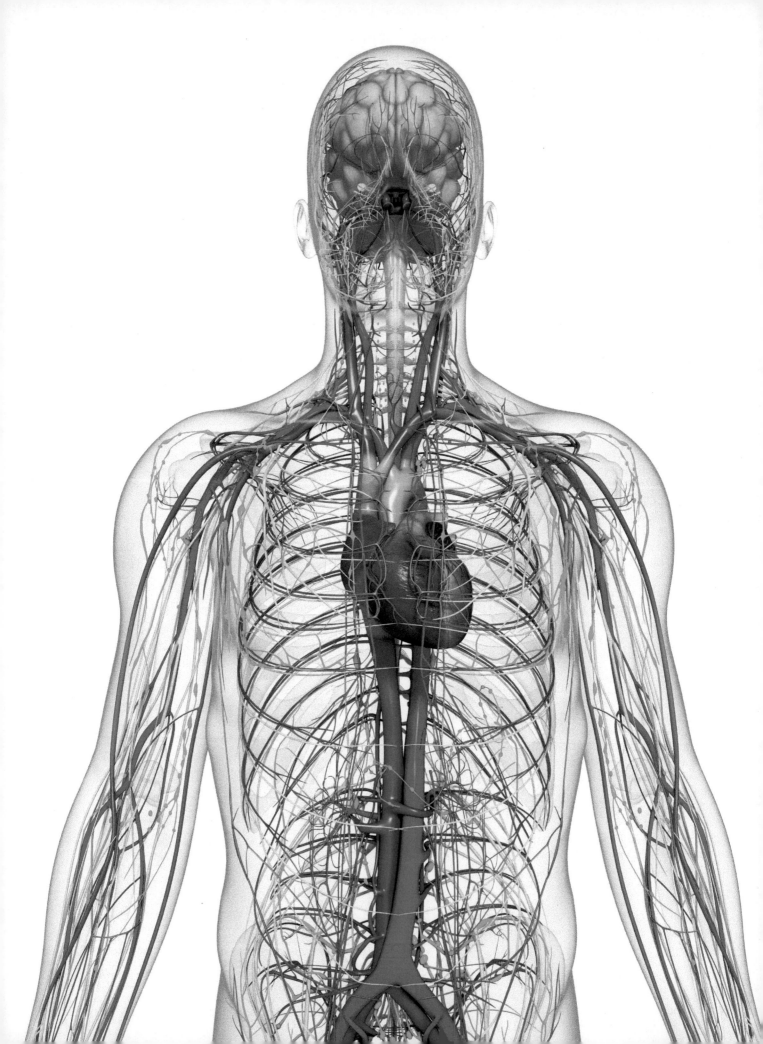

The male reproductive system

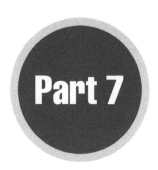

Part 7

Chapters

36 The external male genitalia

Figure 36.1   The left testis and epididymis.

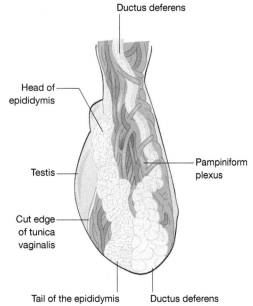

- Ductus deferens
- Head of epididymis
- Testis
- Cut edge of tunica vaginalis
- Pampiniform plexus
- Tail of the epididymis
- Ductus deferens

Source: Heffner L & Schust D. The Reproductive System at a Glance, 4e (2014).

Figure 36.2   Sagittal view of the penis and male pelvis.

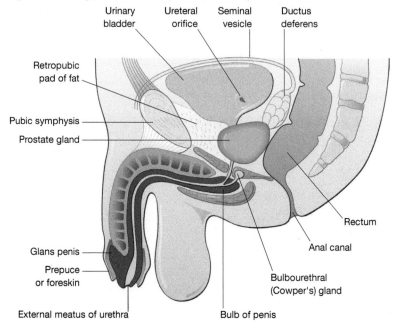

- Urinary bladder
- Ureteral orifice
- Seminal vesicle
- Ductus deferens
- Retropubic pad of fat
- Pubic symphysis
- Prostate gland
- Glans penis
- Prepuce or foreskin
- External meatus of urethra
- Rectum
- Anal canal
- Bulbourethral (Cowper's) gland
- Bulb of penis

Source: Heffner L & Schust D. The Reproductive System at a Glance, 4e (2014).

Figure 36.3   The anatomy of the penis.

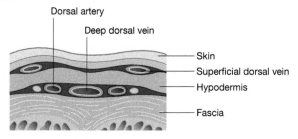

- Dorsal artery
- Deep dorsal vein
- Skin
- Superficial dorsal vein
- Hypodermis
- Fascia

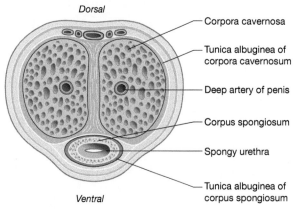

- Dorsal
- Corpora cavernosa
- Tunica albuginea of corpora cavernosum
- Deep artery of penis
- Corpus spongiosum
- Spongy urethra
- Tunica albuginea of corpus spongiosum
- Ventral

Source: Peate I, Wild K & Nair M (eds). Nursing Practice: Knowledge and Care (2014).

Anatomy and Physiology for Nursing and Healthcare Students at a Glance, Second Edition. Ian Peate.
© 2022 John Wiley & Sons Ltd. Published 2022 by John Wiley & Sons Ltd.
Companion website: www.wiley.com/go/peate/anatomyandphysiology

Unlike the female reproductive system, the male reproductive system is more evident as the majority of the organs of the male reproductive system are located externally (Figures 36.1 and 36.2). The prostate gland is discussed in Chapter 37.

The male reproductive system works with other body systems, producing hormones essential for biological development, sexual behaviour and sexual performance. Other body systems include the neuroendocrine system and musculoskeletal system. The male reproductive system is also central to the effective functioning of the urinary system.

The male reproductive system includes the scrotum, testes, spermatic ducts, sex glands and penis. Working together, these organs produce sperm, the male gamete and the other components of semen. They also work together in delivering semen out of the body and into the vagina where it can fertilise egg cells in order to reproduce.

The key functions of the male reproductive system are to:

- produce, maintain and transport the male reproductive cells (sperm) as well as the fluid semen
- ejaculate semen from the penis
- produce and secrete the male sex hormones.

The testes

The reproductive glands of the male are the testes, the male equivalent of the ovaries.

Developmentally, the testes are located in the abdominal cavity of the fetus they descend down through the inguinal canal into the scrotal sac and are suspended on either side of the penis. It is usual for one teste to hang lower than the other. The testes are external to the body. For sperm to be sustainable, it must be produced at a temperature lower than core body temperature, which is why the testes are located in the scrotal sac.

The testes are oval-shaped organs approximately the size of very large olives lying in the scrotal sac, secured and suspended at either end of the spermatic cord. There are usually two testes. Three layers of serous fibrous tissue, the tunica vaginalis, tunica albuginea and tunica vasculosa, surround them.

The testes are responsible for producing testosterone, the primary male sex hormone; they also generate sperm. Within the testes are coiled masses of tubes – the seminiferous tubules. These are responsible for producing the sperm cells through spermatogenesis. There are spaces between the tubules comprising a cluster of cells – the Leydig cells which manufacture and secrete testosterone and other androgens.

Spermatogenesis

Spermatogenesis occurs in the seminiferous tubules of the testes and usually begins around puberty. Starting at puberty, a male will produce millions of sperm every single day for the rest of his life. The seminiferous tubules contain diploid cells – spermatogonia that mature to become sperm. Spermatogenesis turns each one of the diploid spermatogonia into four haploid sperm cells; quadrupling is accomplished through meiotic cell division.

During interphase before meiosis I, the spermatogonium's 46 single chromosomes are duplicated to form 46 pairs of sister chromatids, which exchange genetic material before the first meiotic division. In meiosis II, the two daughter cells will divide and again will produce four cells containing a unique set of 23 single chromosomes that eventually develop into four sperm cells. The sperm

are released from the Sertoli cells entering the lumen of the seminiferous tubules and are pushed along the various ducts within the testes.

The penis

The penis is the male organ for sexual intercourse. It is composed of three parts: the root, attached to the wall of the abdomen; the body or shaft; and the glans at the end of the penis. The glans (when present) is covered with a loose layer of skin, the foreskin. The opening of the urethra transports semen and urine, at the tip of the glans penis. The penis contains a number of sensitive nerve endings and is highly vascular.

The body is cylindrical, consisting of three internal chambers, made up of special, sponge-like erectile tissue, containing thousands of large spaces that fill with blood when sexually aroused (Figure 36.3). As it fills with blood, the penis becomes rigid and erect, allowing for sexual penetration. Penile skin is loose and elastic, accommodating changes in penis size during an erection. When the penile compartments fill with blood, parasympathetic nervous system arteriolar vasodilation occurs. The erection reflex is prompted by sight, sound, smell, touch, pressure or visual stimulation. After ejaculation, vasoconstriction of the arterioles occurs and the penis becomes flaccid.

The epididymis

A long, coiled tube that rests on the back of each testicle, the epididymis transports and stores sperm cells produced in the testes. The epididymis brings sperm to maturity, as sperm leaving the testes are immature and unable to fertilise the egg.

Vas deferens, ejaculatory ducts and spermatic cord

The vas deferens is a long, muscular tube that travels from the epididymis into the pelvic cavity behind the bladder, transporting mature sperm to the urethra ready for ejaculation. The ejaculatory ducts are formed by the fusion of the vas deferens and the seminal vesicles, emptying into the urethra. The seminal vesicles are sac-like pouches that are attached to the vas deferens close to the base of the bladder, producing a fructose-rich fluid that provides the sperm with a source of energy and assisting also with sperm motility.

Clinical practice point

Erectile dysfunction is the inability to achieve and maintain an erection and is a common condition in older men. There are a range of causes of erectile dysfunction, which can be both physical and psychological. Physical causes include a narrowing of the blood vessels to the penis (this is commonly associated with hypertension), hypercholesterolaemia or diabetes mellitus, hormonal problems, surgery or trauma. The psychological causes of erectile dysfunction include anxiety, depression and relational problems. Occasionally erectile dysfunction only occurs in specific situations. The person may be able to get an erection during masturbation, or they may find that they sometimes wake up with an erection, for example, but they are unable to get an erection with their sexual partner. If this does occur, the underlying cause of erectile dysfunction is likely to be psychological (stress related). If the person is unable to get an erection under any circumstances, it is likely that the underlying cause will be physical. Erectile dysfunction can also be a side-effect of using certain medicines.

37 The prostate gland

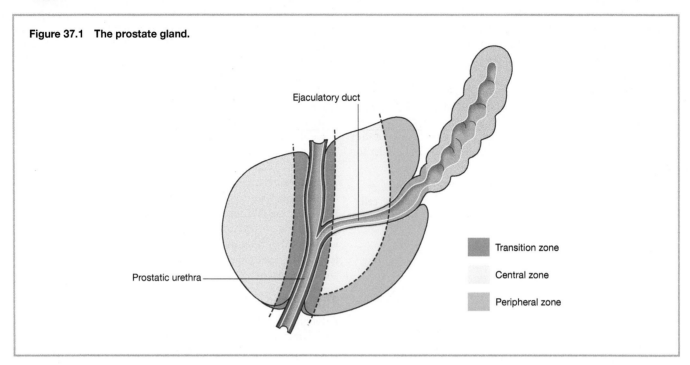

Figure 37.1 The prostate gland.

Ejaculatory duct

Prostatic urethra

Transition zone

Central zone

Peripheral zone

Anatomy and Physiology for Nursing and Healthcare Students at a Glance, Second Edition. Ian Peate.
© 2022 John Wiley & Sons Ltd. Published 2022 by John Wiley & Sons Ltd.
Companion website: www.wiley.com/go/peate/anatomyandphysiology

Not all the functions of the prostate gland are fully understood. The prostate is an exocrine gland and part of the male reproductive system, It is the largest accessory gland in the male reproductive system.

A layer of fibrous tissue called the prostatic capsule covers the prostate gland. A thin layer of connective tissue separates the prostate and seminal vesicles from the rectum posteriorly.

The prostate gland is made up of a number of different types of cells:

- gland cells that produce the fluid portion of semen
- muscle cells that control urine flow and ejaculation
- fibrous cells that provide the supportive structure of the gland.

The prostate is a firm gland; it is partly glandular and has a partly muscular body, located immediately below the internal urethral orifice and around the beginning aspect of the urethra. It is located in the pelvic cavity, below the lower part of the symphysis pubis, above the superior fascia of the urogenital diaphragm and in front of the rectum. It is about the size of a chestnut and somewhat conical in shape with three zones (Figure 37.1).

Arterial blood supply to the prostate is derived from branches of the internal iliac artery. Venous blood collects in the periprostatic venous plexus from where it is returned to the internal iliac vein by the inferior vesical vein.

Lymphatics from the prostate typically travel to internal iliac nodes, including the more anterior group of obturator nodes.

The prostate receives an autonomic nerve supply from the inferior hypogastric plexus, which lies along the internal iliac artery.

Zones of the prostate gland

Peripheral zone

The peripheral zone of the prostate gland is the area that is closest to the rectum. It is the largest zone of the prostate gland and accounts for 70% of the total gland.

Transition zone

The transition zone is the middle area of the prostate, located between the peripheral and central zones. It surrounds the urethra as it passes through the prostate. Up until the age of around 40 years, this zone makes up approximately 20% of the prostate gland. As a man ages, the transition zone begins to enlarge, until it becomes the largest area of the prostate. As the transition zone enlarges, it pushes the peripheral zone of the prostate toward the rectum.

Central zone

The central zone is situated in front of the transition zone. This zone is farthest from the rectum and it contains approximately one-third of the ducts that secrete fluid that help to create semen.

Surfaces of the prostate gland

The gland has a number of surfaces:

- a base
- an apex
- an anterior
- a posterior
- two lateral surfaces.

Base

The base on palpation is directed upwards and inferior to the surface of the bladder. The urethra penetrates it closer to its anterior border than its posterior border.

Apex

The apex is small and is directed downwards and in contact with the urogenital diaphragm. The urethra exits through the apex.

Anterior, inferolateral and posterior surfaces

The anterior surface is narrow and is connected with the puboprostatic ligament. The paired inferolateral surfaces, which are separated from the levator ani by the prostatic venous plexus, curve inwards both anteriorly and inferiorly. The posterior surface is broad, narrows inferiorly and can be defined by a shallow longitudinal depression into the right and left sides. The ejaculatory ducts join the prostate near the superior extent of this ridge.

Function of the prostate gland

Prostatic fluid

The key function of the prostate gland (which is regulated by the hormone testosterone) is to produce the fluid aspect of semen. This assists with sperm motility and survival by providing a protective and fluid medium for the passage of semen through the vagina for fertilisation. The gland cells within the prostate produce a thin alkaline fluid that is rich in proteins and minerals, maintaining and nourishing the sperm. This fluid is continually produced but when the man is sexually aroused, the prostate gland produces larger amounts of prostatic fluid. It then mixes with sperm and this is then ejaculated as semen.

The prostate also controls the flow of urine. The muscle fibres of the gland are wrapped around the urethra under involuntary nervous system control. These fibres contract to slow and stop the flow of urine.

Some structures around the prostate gland

- *Seminal vesicles* – these glands produce semen and are located on both sides of the prostate.
- *Vas deferens* – these tubes carry sperm from the testicles to the seminal vesicles.
- *Nerve bundles* – these control bladder and erectile function and are located on both sides of the prostate.
- *Muscles* – control urination.

Prostate specific antigen

Prostate specific antigen (PSA) is a fluid produced in the prostate which plays a key role in enabling sperm to travel into the uterus by preserving the semen in liquid form. PSA is produced exclusively by epithelial prostatic cells. It counteracts the clotting enzyme in the seminal vesicle fluid, which principally glues the semen to the cervix, located next to the uterine entrance inside the vagina. PSA dissolves this enzyme with its own enzyme in order to permit the sperm to enter the uterus and fertilise an egg.

Clinical practice point

A digital rectal examination is used to examine the prostate to determine if the person may have a prostate problem or prostate cancer. It involves a nurse or doctor palpating the prostate gland through the wall of the rectum. The examination may be undertaken in a hospital, clinic or GP surgery. The patient is asked to lie on his side on an examination table, with his knees brought up towards his chest. A gloved lubricated finger is gently inserted into the rectum. The examination is not usually painful and does not take long to perform. Some people can find the procedure slightly uncomfortable or embarrassing. The results of the examination may reveal a prostate gland that is normal (normal size for the person's age with a smooth surface), larger than expected for the person's age (this might be a sign of an enlarged prostate) or hard or lumpy (this may be a sign of prostate cancer). A digital rectal examination is not a completely accurate test as it is the peripheral zone of the prostate that is mainly palpated during the examination. The results of the examination are sent to the person's GP. The GP will discuss the results and explain what they mean.

38 Spermatogenesis

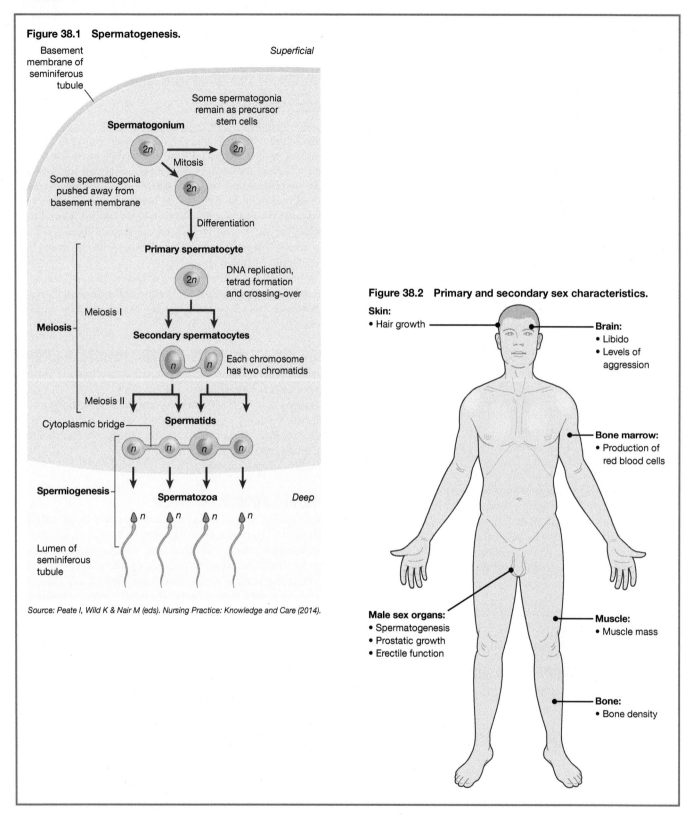

Figure 38.1   Spermatogenesis.

Basement membrane of seminiferous tubule

Superficial

Spermatogonium

Some spermatogonia remain as precursor stem cells

2n → 2n

Mitosis

Some spermatogonia pushed away from basement membrane

2n

Differentiation

Primary spermatocyte

2n

DNA replication, tetrad formation and crossing-over

Meiosis

Meiosis I

Secondary spermatocytes

n   n

Each chromosome has two chromatids

Meiosis II

Cytoplasmic bridge

Spermatids

n   n   n   n

Spermiogenesis

Spermatozoa

Deep

n   n   n   n

Lumen of seminiferous tubule

Source: Peate I, Wild K & Nair M (eds). Nursing Practice: Knowledge and Care (2014).

Figure 38.2   Primary and secondary sex characteristics.

Skin:
• Hair growth

Brain:
• Libido
• Levels of aggression

Bone marrow:
• Production of red blood cells

Male sex organs:
• Spermatogenesis
• Prostatic growth
• Erectile function

Muscle:
• Muscle mass

Bone:
• Bone density

Anatomy and Physiology for Nursing and Healthcare Students at a Glance, Second Edition. Ian Peate.
© 2022 John Wiley & Sons Ltd. Published 2022 by John Wiley & Sons Ltd.
Companion website: www.wiley.com/go/peate/anatomyandphysiology

The process by which the spermatogonia (male primordial germ cells) undergo meiosis to produce a number of spermatozoa is called spermatogenesis. This process commences at puberty, continuing for as long as the man lives, as opposed to oogenesis (production of the primordial ova), which occurs only during fetal life. Males begin to produce sperm when they reach puberty, usually from 10 to 16 years old. Males continually produce sperm in large quantities (about 200 million a day). This large production maximises the likelihood of sperm reaching the egg following ejaculation.

The process by which male primary sperm cells undergo meiosis is called spermatogenesis and this results in the production of a number of cells termed spermatogonia, from which the primary spermatocytes are derived. Each primary spermatocyte divides into two secondary spermatocytes and each secondary spermatocyte into two spermatids or young spermatozoa. These develop into mature spermatozoa, also known as sperm cells.

Spermatogenesis occurs in the seminiferous tubules of the testes (Figure 38.1). Diploid (46 chromosome) germ cells known as spermatogonia line the basement membrane of each seminiferous tubule. The spermatogonia move away from the basement membrane as meiosis occurs; as they mature they become primary spermatocytes. Meiosis occurs again and this produces two haploid (23 chromosome) cells called secondary spermatocytes. Four spermatids are the result of the two secondary spermatocytes undergoing meiosis.

For spermatids to develop into sperm, this is dependent on the Sertoli cells present in the seminiferous tubules. Attaching themselves to the Sertoli cells, the spermatids receive the nourishment needed and the hormonal signals required to develop into sperm.

It takes approximately 70–80 days for spermatogenesis to occur – from meiotic division of a spermatogonium to the maturation of a mature spermatid. The mature sperm travel from the seminiferous tubules to the epididymis. While the sperm are fully mature by the time they are ejaculated, they do not become motile until they are activated by biochemicals in the semen and in the female reproductive tract.

Semen is a white or grey liquid that is discharged from the urethra on ejaculation. Usually, each millilitre of semen contains millions of spermatozoa, but the majority of the volume is made up of secretions of the glands in the male reproductive organs.

Sperm will only survive in warm environments. As the sperm leave the body, their survival is reduced and this may cause the cells to die, which decreases the quality of the sperm.

There are two types of sperm cells: 'male' and 'female'. Those sperm cells that give rise to female (XX) offspring after fertilisation carry an X chromosome, while sperm cells that give rise to male (XY) offspring only carry a Y chromosome.

The sperm cell is made up of a head, midpiece and tail. The head contains the nucleus containing densely coiled chromatin fibres, surrounded anteriorly by an acrosome, which contains enzymes that are used for penetrating the female egg. The midpiece has a central filamentous core with a number of mitochondria spiralled around it, used for adenosine triphosphate (ATP) production required for the journey through the female cervix, uterus and uterine tubes. The tail or 'flagellum' performs the lashing movements needed to propel the spermatocyte.

Male sex hormones

The major female and male hormones can be classified as oestrogens or androgens. Both classes of male and female hormones are present in both males and females alike, but differ vastly in their amounts.

Testosterone is the primary male sex hormone; it is a steroid that regulates growth and development. Testosterone production increases exponentially (approximately 18-fold) during puberty.

It is usual after puberty for the interstitial cells to produce testosterone continually. Approximately 6 mg of testosterone is produced each day. Testosterone production may be disrupted for a number of reasons. Once a man reaches 40 years of age, testosterone production declines; on average men experience a 1% per year drop in testosterone production once they reach this age.

Testosterone functions to develop a man's primary and secondary sex characteristics (Figure 38.2). Primary sex characteristics include size of penis and testes size in adult men – testosterone is responsible for developing the male genitals, spermatogenesis and regulating libido. Erectile function is influenced by testosterone as this increases the activity of nitric oxide synthase which regulates the movement of smooth muscles in the penis. Increased nitric oxide synthase activity increases relaxation of smooth muscles in the penis, improving the ability to achieve and maintain an erection.

Secondary sex characteristics include the growth of hair (pubic, body and facial hair), a deep voice and heavier bones. Greater quantities of testosterone cause men to have a greater proportion of lean body mass and lower proportion of fat compared to women.

When the male reaches puberty, there is an increase in the secretion of gonadotrophin-releasing hormone (GnRH) from the hypothalamus. GnRH then stimulates the anterior aspect of the pituitary gland to increase secretion of luteinising hormone (LH) and follicle stimulating hormone (FSH); this negative feedback mechanism controls secretion of testosterone and spermatogenesis.

The Leydig cells (located between seminiferous tubules) are stimulated by LH to secrete testosterone; testosterone is synthesised from cholesterol in the testes. The Leydig cells produce 95% of a man's testosterone. Through negative feedback, the secretion of LH is suppressed by the anterior pituitary and secretion of GnRH is suppressed by the hypothalamus. Testosterone in some target cells, for example in the prostate gland, is converted to dihydrotestosterone (DHT).

FSH indirectly acts to stimulate spermatogenesis, with FSH and testosterone acting synergistically on the Sertoli cells to stimulate discharge of androgen-binding protein (ABP) into the lumen of the seminiferous tubules as well as the interstitial fluid surrounding the spermatogenic cells. ABP attaches to testosterone, keeping the concentration high. Testosterone is responsible for stimulating the final steps of spermatogenesis in the seminiferous tubules.

Sertoli cells release inhibin (a hormone). Once the degree of spermatogenesis required for male reproduction functions has been achieved, inhibin inhibits FSH secretion by the anterior pituitary gland. Less inhibin is released when spermatogenesis is happening too slowly and as such, more FHS is produced, resulting in an increased rate of spermatogenesis

Clinical practice point

A low sperm count, also called oligozoospermia, is where a man has fewer than 15 million sperm per millilitre of semen. Problems with sperm, including a low sperm count and problems with sperm quality, are common. They are a factor in around 1 in 3 couples who are struggling to get pregnant. There are treatments available that can help a man become a father if he has a low sperm count. It is not always obvious what is causing a low sperm count. Sometimes problems with sperm count and quality are associated with a hormone imbalance, such as hypogonadism, a genetic problem such as Klinefelter syndrome, having had undescended testes as a baby, damage to the sperm-producing structures, genital infection (for example, chlamydia, gonorrhoea, prostatitis), varicocoeles, previous surgery to the testes, the testes becoming overheated, excessive alcohol consumption, smoking and using drugs such as marijuana or cocaine, being overweight or obese. Some medications can also result in problems with sperm count.

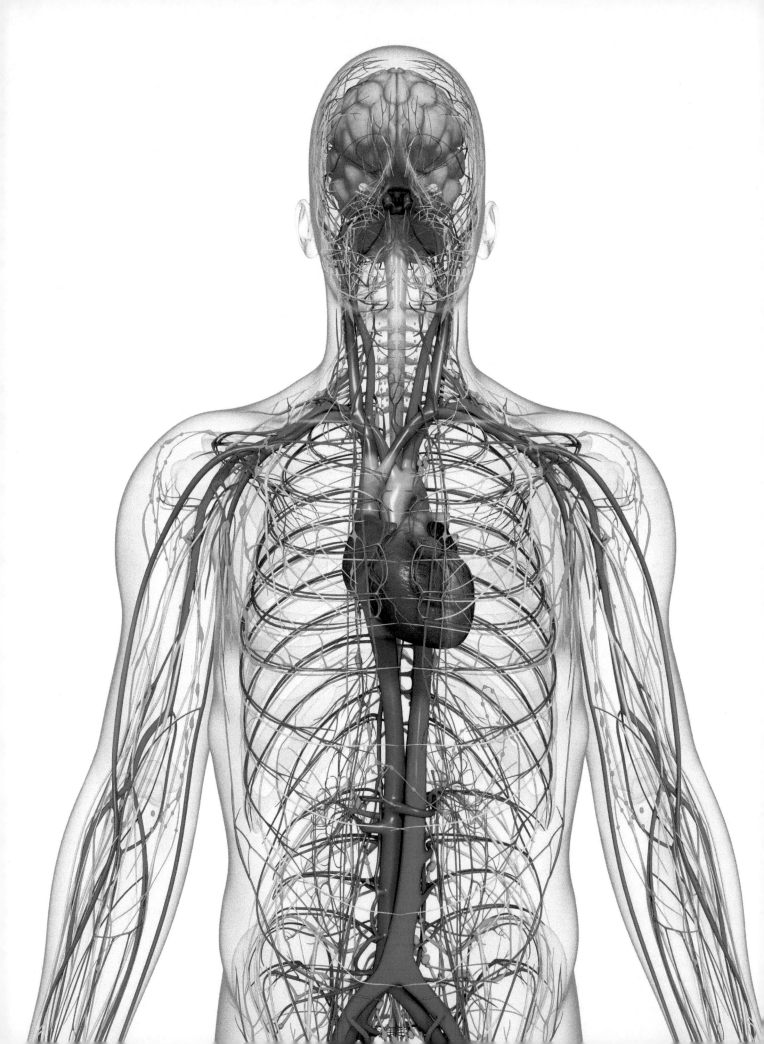

The female reproductive system

Part 8

Chapters

39 The female internal reproductive organs

Figure 39.1 The female reproductive organs.

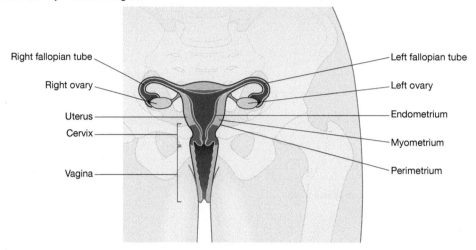

Right fallopian tube
Right ovary
Uterus
Cervix
Vagina

Left fallopian tube
Left ovary
Endometrium
Myometrium
Perimetrium

Table 39.1 The layers of the uterus.

Layer	Comments
The perimetrium	A serous membrane that envelopes the uterus, the outer layer; provides support to the uterus located within the pelvis. Also known as the parietal peritoneum.
The myometrium	The middle layer made up of smooth muscle. Throughout pregnancy and childbirth the uterus has to stretch and the muscular layer permits this to occur. The muscle will contact during labour and post natally this muscular layer contracts forcefully to force out the placenta.
The endometrium	The inner layer of the uterus with a mucus lining. The exterior is continuous with the vagina and the fallopian tubes. During menstruation the layers of the endometrium are shed, sloughing away from the inner layer, this is the menstrual period occurring as a result of hormonal changes taking place. The endometrium thickens during the menstrual period becoming rich with blood vessels and glandular tissue until the next period occurs and the cycle begins again.

Anatomy and Physiology for Nursing and Healthcare Students at a Glance, Second Edition. Ian Peate.
© 2022 John Wiley & Sons Ltd. Published 2022 by John Wiley & Sons Ltd.
Companion website: www.wiley.com/go/peate/anatomyandphysiology

The female reproduction system produces the female egg cells (called the ova or oocytes) which are essential for reproduction and the female sex hormones that maintain the reproductive cycle. This system is both a reproductive system as well as containing the female sex organs.

Internal female reproductive organs

The female internal sex organs consist of the ovaries, fallopian tubes, uterus and vagina (Figure 39.1).

Ovaries

The ovaries are the primary reproductive organs as well as producing female sex hormones; they are paired glands. In the adult woman, they are flat, almond-shaped structures situated on each side of the uterus beneath the ends of the fallopian tubes. Ligaments hold them in position, attaching them to the uterus; they are also attached to the broad ligament, and this ligament attaches them to the pelvic wall. The ovaries provide a space for storage of the female germ cells and also produce the female hormones oestrogen and progesterone. A woman's total number of ova is present at her birth. When a girl reaches puberty she usually ovulates each month.

The ovary contains a number of small structures called ovarian follicles. Each follicle contains an immature ovum (an oocyte). Follicles are stimulated each month by two hormones – follicle-stimulating hormone (FSH) and luteinising hormone (LH); these stimulate the follicles to mature. The developing follicles are enclosed in layers of follicle cells. mature follicles are called graafian follicles.

Ovarian cortex

This lies deep and close to the tunica albuginea containing the ovarian follicles surrounded by dense irregular connective tissue. These follicles contain oocytes in different stages of development and a number of cells that feed the developing oocyte. As the follicle grows, it secretes oestrogen.

Graafian follicles

The graafian follicles manufacture oestrogen, stimulating growth of the endometrium. Each month in the woman who is menstruating, one or two of the mature graafian follicles release an oocyte in what is known as ovulation. The large ruptured follicle becomes a new structure – the corpus luteum, the remnants of a mature follicle.

Corpus luteum

The corpus luteum produces oestrogen and progesterone to support the endometrium until conception or the cycle begins again. The corpus luteum gradually disintegrates; a scar is left on the outside of the ovary (the corpus albicans). The outer ovary is enveloped in a fibrous capsule called the tunica albuginea, composed of cuboidal epithelium. The inner ovary is divided into parts.

Ovarian medulla

The ovarian medulla contains blood vessels, nerves and lymphatic tissues surrounded by loose connective tissue.

Oogenesis

This relates to the development of relatively undifferentiated germ cells – oogonia – which are fixed to between 2–4 million diploid (2n) stem cells during foetal development. All ova are ultimately derived from these clones as they develop into larger primary oocytes; the meiotic phase is not completed until puberty. Every month from puberty until menopause, FSH and LH are released by the anterior pituitary gland, stimulating the primordial follicles; only one usually reaches the maturity needed for ovulation.

Female sex hormones

The ovaries produce oestrogens, progesterone and androgens recurrently. Oestrogens are essential for the development and maintenance of secondary sex characteristics working with a number of other hormones, stimulating the female reproductive system to prepare for the growth of a fetus and playing a key role in the normal structure of the skin and blood vessels. These hormones help reduce the rate of bone resorption, enhance increased high-density lipoproteins, decrease cholesterol levels and increase blood clotting.

The uterus

This is a hollow muscular organ in the pelvic cavity posterior and superior to the urinary bladder, anterior to the rectum, approximately 7.5 cm long. The fundus is a thick muscular region above the fallopian tubes; the body is joined to the cervix by the isthmus. The uterine wall has three distinct layers (Table 39.1).

The fallopian tubes

The paired fallopian tubes are delicate, thin cylindrical structures approximately 8–14 cm long, attached to the uterus on one end supported by the broad ligaments. The lateral ends of the fallopian tubes are open and made of projections called fimbriae draped over the ovary. The fimbriae pick up the ovum after discharge from the ovary; they are composed of smooth muscle lined with ciliated mucus-producing epithelial cells, transporting the ovum along the tubes towards the uterus. Fertilisation of the ovum usually occurs in the outer portion of the fallopian tubes.

The vagina

A tubular, fibromuscular structure approximately 8–10 cm in length, the vagina is the receptacle for the penis during sexual intercourse. It is an organ of sexual response, while the canal also allows menstrual flow to leave the body and is the passage for the birth of the child. It is situated posterior to the urinary bladder and urethra, anterior to the rectum. The upper element houses the uterine cervix. Vaginal walls are made of membranous folds of rugae, composed of mucus-secreting stratified squamous epithelial cells.

Usually the vaginal walls are moist with a pH ranging from 3.8 to 4.2. Oestrogen causes the growth of vaginal mucosal cells, thickening and developing them, increasing glycogen content and resulting in a slight acidification of the vaginal fluid.

The cervix

The cervix forms a pathway between the uterus and the vagina. The uterine opening of the cervix is the internal os and the vaginal opening the external os. The space between these openings, the endocervical canal, acts as a conduit for the discharge of menstrual fluid, the opening for semen and delivery of the infant during birth.

Clinical practice point

Pain during or after sex is known as dyspareunia. It can be caused by a number of things, for example illness, infection, a physical health problem or a psychological health problem. Dyspareunia should not be ignored and help should be sought. Pain during sex can affect both men and women. Women can experience pain during or after sex, either in the vagina or deeper in the pelvis. Vaginal pain could be caused by *Candida*, a sexually transmitted infection, the menopause, lack of sexual arousal, vaginismus (a condition where muscles in or around the vagina squeeze shut or go into spasm), genital irritation or allergy. When the woman feels pain inside the pelvis, this can be caused by conditions such as pelvic inflammatory disease, endometriosis, fibroids, irritable bowel syndrome or constipation.

40 The external female genitalia

Figure 40.1 The external female genitalia.

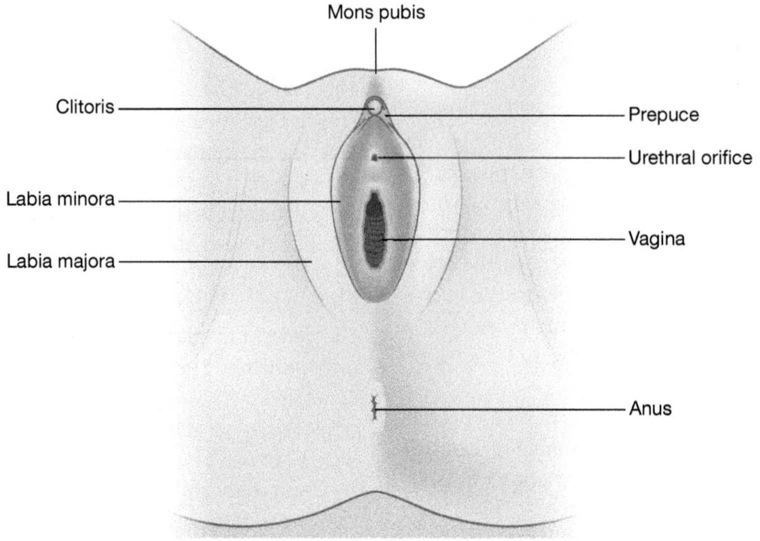

Mons pubis

Clitoris —————— Prepuce

————— Urethral orifice

Labia minora —————— Vagina

Labia majora —————

————— Anus

The external female genitalia are known collectively as the vulva. They include the mons pubis, labia, clitoris, vaginal and urethral openings, and glands (Figure 40.1). The external genitalia have three key functions.

- Enabling sperm to enter the body.
- Protecting the internal genital organs from infectious organisms.
- The provision of sexual pleasure.

Mons veneris

Mons veneris is Latin for 'hill of Venus' (Venus was the Roman goddess of love); it is the pad of elevated fatty tissue that covers the pubic bone situated inferior to the abdomen and superior to the labia. The amount of fat increases during puberty and decreases after the menopause. The mons acts to protect the pubic bone from the impact of sexual intercourse. During puberty, the mons is covered with coarse pubic hair, after puberty this decreases.

Labia majora

These are the outer lips of the vulva and they are made of two symmetrical pads of fatty tissue that wrap around the vulva, extending from the mons to the perineum. They provide protection for the urethral and vaginal openings. It is usual for these labia to be covered with pubic hair; they contain a number of sweat and oil glands and the scent (pheromones) from these glands may have a role to play in sexual arousal.

Labia minora

The inner lips of the vulva, known as the labia minora, are composed of thin stretches of tissue within the labia majora, folding and protecting the vagina, urethra and clitoris. They are thin, delicate folds of fat-free hairless skin located between the labia majora. The labia minora contain a core of spongy tissue within which there are many small blood vessels but no fat. The appearance of the labia minora varies from woman to woman, from tiny lips that are hidden between the labia majora to larger lips that can protrude. Internally, the surface consists of thin skin and has a pink colour associated with mucous membranes. It contains a number of sensory nerve endings. Both the inner and outer labia are very sensitive to touch and pressure.

Clitoris

The clitoris is a small body of spongy tissue located at the top of the labia minora and is highly sexually sensitive. Externally, it is only the tip or glans of the clitoris that is visible; the organ itself is elongated and branches into two forks, the crura, which then extend downwards along the edge of the vaginal opening toward the perineum. On average, the clitoris is approximately 3 cm in length. The external tip of the clitoris or the clitoral glans is protected by the prepuce (also called the clitoral hood), a covering of tissue that is analogous to the foreskin of the male penis. The clitoris can extend and the hood retracts to make the clitoral glans more accessible during sexual excitement. The clitoris is an erectile organ and is usually hidden by the labia when flaccid.

The clitoris will, like the penis, enlarge upon tactile stimulation; it does not, however, lengthen significantly. It is highly sensitive and very important in the sexual arousal of a female. There are variations in size and the clitoral glans may be very small in some women while others may have a large clitoris and the hood may not completely cover it. The clitoris is suspended by a suspensory ligament.

Urethra

The external urethral orifice is located 2–3 cm posterior to the clitoris and immediately anterior to the vaginal orifice. The openings of the ducts of the paraurethral glands (also called Skene's glands) are situated on each side of the vaginal orifice. These glands are homologous to the male prostate gland. The urethra is not related to sex or reproduction; it is where urine is excreted when it is passed from the urinary bladder.

Hymen

The hymen is a thin pinkish membrane found at the lower end of the vagina. it is often shaped like a crescent, though there may be many other forms. In nearly all young women, there is a large gap in the membrane. In other words, it does not block off the vagina completely. This is important, because the hole in the hymen allows menstrual blood to come through when the girl starts her periods. The hymen is the traditional symbol of virginity; as it is a very thin membrane, it can be torn by vigorous exercise, insertion of a tampon, masturbation or the use of sex toys such as dildos.

Blood supply

Arterial supply

The rich arterial supply to the vulva comes from two external pudendal arteries as well as one internal pudendal artery located on either side. The internal pudendal artery supplies the skin, sex organs and perineal muscles. The labial arteries are branches of the internal pudendal artery and this is the same for the dorsal and deep arteries of the clitoris.

Venous drainage

The veins of the pelvis drain deoxygenated blood and then return it to the heart. There are three major vessels involved in venous drainage of the pelvis: the external iliac vein, internal iliac vein and common iliac vein (these correspond to the major pelvic arteries).

Lymphatic drainage

Within the vulva there are a number of very rich networks of lymphatic channels. The majority of lymph vessels pass to the superficial inguinal lymph nodes and deep inguinal nodes.

Nerve supply

The nerves that supply the vulva are branches of the:

- ilioinguinal nerve
- genital branch of the genitofemoral nerve
- perineal branch of the femoral cutaneous nerve
- perineal nerve.

Clinical practice point

Female genital mutilation (FGM) is a procedure where the female genitals are deliberately cut, injured or changed, but there is no medical reason for this to be carried out (it is also known as female circumcision or cutting, and by other terms such as sunna, gudniin, halalays, tahur, megrez and khitan). FGM is usually carried out on young girls between infancy and the age of 15 years, most commonly undertaken before puberty begins. FGM is illegal in the UK and is classified as child abuse. This very painful act can seriously harm the health of women and girls. It can also result in long-term problems with sex, childbirth and mental health. There are four main types of FGM: type 1 (clitoridectomy) – removing part or all of the clitoris, type 2 (excision) – removing part or all of the clitoris as well as the inner labia, with or without removal of the labia majora; type 3 (infibulation) – narrowing the vaginal opening by creating a seal, formed by cutting and repositioning the labia; type 4 – other harmful procedures to the female genitals, including pricking, piercing, cutting, scraping or burning the area.

41 The female breast

Figure 41.1 The breast.

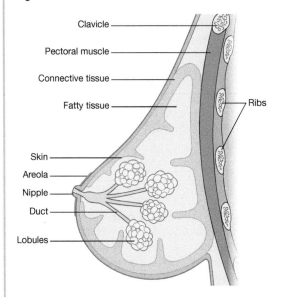

- Clavicle
- Pectoral muscle
- Connective tissue
- Fatty tissue
- Ribs
- Skin
- Areola
- Nipple
- Duct
- Lobules

Figure 41.2 The breast and surrounding structures.

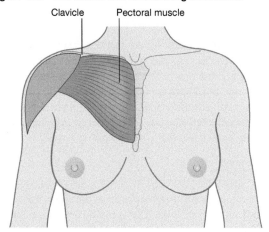

- Clavicle
- Pectoral muscle

Figure 41.3 Lobules and ducts.

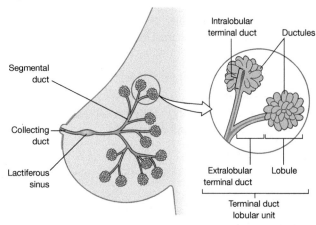

- Segmental duct
- Collecting duct
- Lactiferous sinus
- Intralobular terminal duct
- Ductules
- Extralobular terminal duct
- Lobule
- Terminal duct lobular unit

Figure 41.4 The axillary lymph nodes.

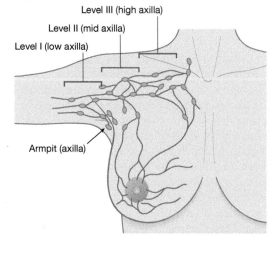

- Level III (high axilla)
- Level II (mid axilla)
- Level I (low axilla)
- Armpit (axilla)

Figure 41.5 Breast lymph.

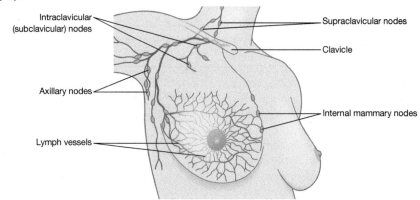

- Intraclavicular (subclavicular) nodes
- Supraclavicular nodes
- Clavicle
- Axillary nodes
- Internal mammary nodes
- Lymph vessels

Anatomy and Physiology for Nursing and Healthcare Students at a Glance, Second Edition. Ian Peate.
© 2022 John Wiley & Sons Ltd. Published 2022 by John Wiley & Sons Ltd.
Companion website: www.wiley.com/go/peate/anatomyandphysiology

The female breast is a part of the female external reproductive system. It contains the mammary glands which are key structures involved in lactation. Women have more breast tissue than men.

The female breast

Function

The key function of the breast is to produce, store and release milk to feed a baby. Milk is produced in lobules located throughout the breast after they have been stimulated by hormones when the woman has given birth. The milk is carried to the nipple by the ducts and from the nipple to the baby during breastfeeding.

Structure

The structure of the female breast is complex. Within it there is fat and connective tissue, as well as lobes, lobules, ducts and lymph nodes (Figure 41.1). The breast lies over a muscle of the chest known as the pectoral muscle. The female breast covers a large area; it extends from just below the collarbone (clavicle), to the armpit (axilla) and across to the breastbone (sternum) (Figure 41.2). The breast is a mass of glandular, fatty and connective tissue.

Lobules and ducts

Each breast contains a number of lobules (sections) that branch out from the nipple; the lobules are the glands that produce the milk. A lobule holds tiny, hollow alveoli linked by a network of thin ducts (Figure 41.3). During breastfeeding, the ducts carry milk from the alveoli toward the breast areola (the dark area of skin in the centre of the breast). From the areola, the ducts join together into larger ducts that terminate at the nipple. The areola (pink or brown in colour) is the circular area around the nipple; this contains small sweat glands which secrete moisture, which acts as a lubricant during breastfeeding. The nipple is the area at the centre of the areola where the milk emerges.

Fat, ligaments and connective tissue

The spaces around the lobules and ducts are filled with fat, ligaments and connective tissue. The amount of fat in the breast determines their size; the fat gives shape to the breast. In all women, the actual milk-producing structures are nearly the same. Cyclical changes in hormone levels have an impact on breast tissue. It is usual for younger women to have denser and less fatty breast tissue than older women who have gone through the menopause. Ligaments provide support to the breast. They run from the skin through the breast, attaching to muscles on the chest.

Nerve supply

There are a number of major nerves located in the breast area, including nerves in the chest and arm. There are also sensory nerves in the skin of the chest and axilla. Branches from the 4th, 5th and 6th thoracic nerves supply the breasts.

Arteries and veins

Arterial blood supply to the breast comes from the thoracic branches of the axillary arteries and the internal mammary and intercostal arteries. Venous drainage of the breast is primarily accomplished by the axillary vein. The subclavian, intercostal and internal thoracic veins also aid in returning the blood to the heart.

Lymph nodes and lymph ducts

The lymphatic system is a network of lymph nodes and ducts that help to fight infection (Figure 41.4). Axillary lymph nodes are located above the clavicle, behind the sternum, as well as in other parts of the body. Lymph circulates throughout body tissues, picking up fats, bacteria and other unwanted materials and filtering them out through the lymphatic system. Breast lymph nodes include the supraclavicular nodes – above the clavicle; infraclavicular (or subclavicular) nodes – below the clavicle; axillary nodes – in the axilla; and internal mammary nodes – inside the chest around the sternum.

There are about 30–50 lymph nodes in the axilla. This number varies from woman to woman. The axillary lymph nodes are divided into three levels depending on how close they are to the pectoral muscle on the chest (Figure 41.5).

- Level I (low axilla) – in the lower or bottom aspect of the axilla, along the outside border of the pectoral muscle.
- Level II (mid axilla) – in the middle part of the axilla, under the pectoral muscle.
- Level III (high axilla) – below and near the centre of the clavicle, above the breast area and along the inside border of the pectoral muscle.

Breast development

Breast tissue changes occur during puberty, during the menstrual cycle, during pregnancy and after menopause. Female breasts do not begin growing until puberty; at this time the breasts respond to hormonal changes, predominantly increases in oestrogen and progesterone. During puberty, breast ducts and milk glands grow. The breast skin stretches as the breasts grow, creating a rounded appearance. Younger women tend to have more glandular tissue than older women. Most of the glandular and ductal tissue in older women is replaced with fatty tissue and the breasts become less dense. Ligaments lose their elasticity as the woman ages, causing the breasts to sag.

The size and shape of women's breasts vary considerably. A woman's breasts are rarely the same size; one breast is often slightly larger or smaller, higher or lower or shaped differently than the other.

Hormones and the breast

The main female hormone is oestrogen, which affects female sexual characteristics, such as breast development, and is necessary for reproduction. The ovaries make up most of the oestrogen in a woman's body; a small amount is made by the adrenal glands. Progesterone (the other female sex hormone) is made in the ovaries. Progesterone prepares the uterus for pregnancy and the breasts for producing milk for breastfeeding (lactation). Each month, breast tissue is exposed to cycles of oestrogen and progesterone throughout a woman's child-bearing years. In the first part of the menstrual cycle, oestrogen stimulates the growth of the milk ducts. Progesterone takes over in the second part, stimulating the lobules. Post menopause, the monthly cycle ends although the adrenal glands continue to produce oestrogen and a woman keeps her sexual characteristics.

> **Clinical practice point**
> There's no right or wrong way for a woman to check her breasts. However, it is important to know how the breasts usually look and feel and to be breast aware. If any changes are identified they should be quickly reported to the practice nurse or GP. Every woman's breasts are different in terms of size, shape and consistency, and one breast may be larger than the other. How the breasts feel at different times of the month can change during the menstrual cycle. Some women, for example, have tender and lumpy breasts, particularly near the axilla, around the time of their period. After the menopause, normal breasts can feel softer, less firm and not as lumpy. Look at the breasts and feel each breast and axilla and up to the clavicle. It may be easiest to do this in the shower or bath, by running a soapy hand over each breast and up under each armpit. Also look at the breasts in the mirror, with the arms by the side and also with them raised.

42 The menstrual cycle

Figure 42.1 Hormonal regulation of the changes in the ovary and uterus.

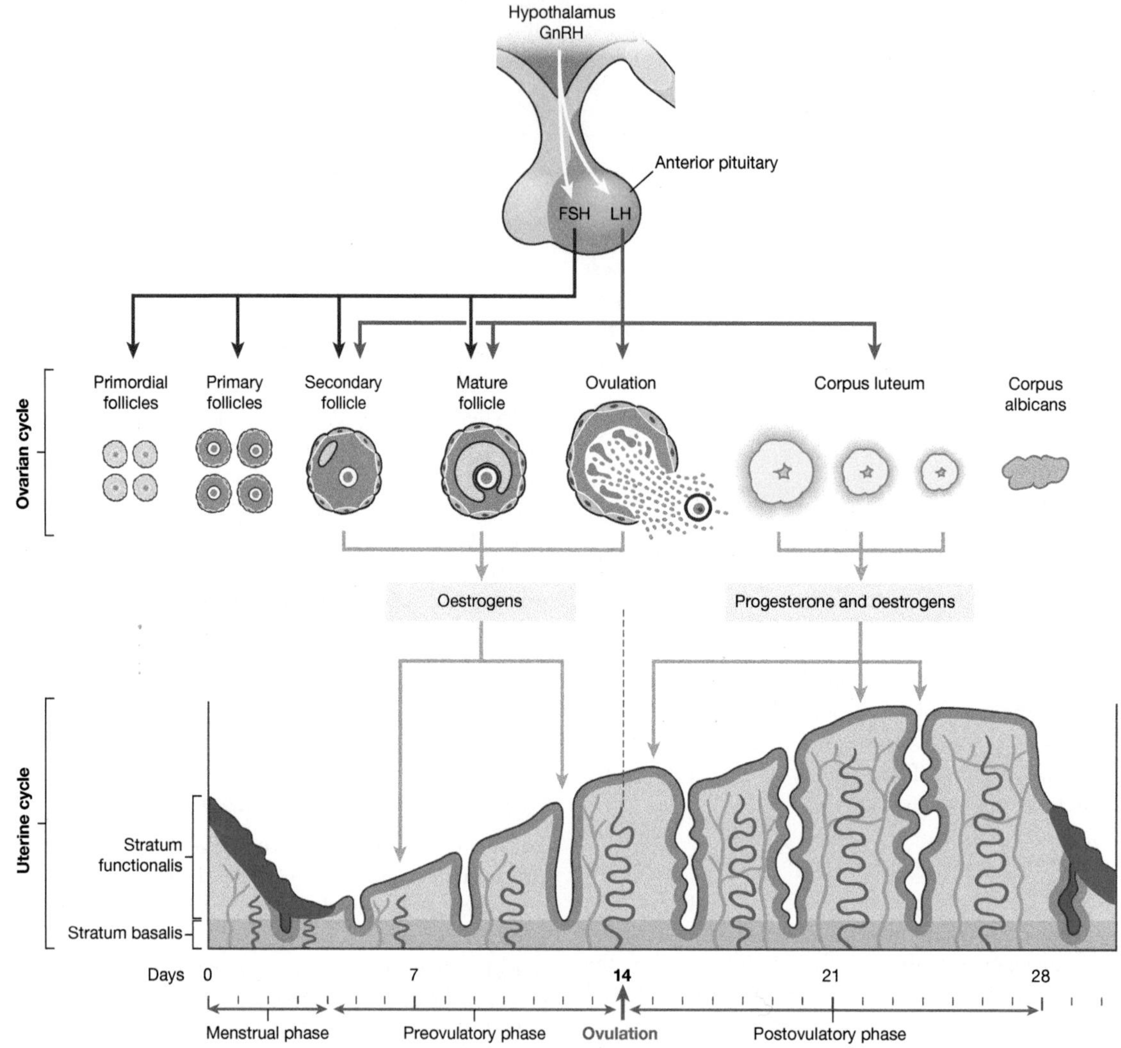

Hypothalamus
GnRH

Anterior pituitary

FSH LH

Ovarian cycle

| Primordial follicles | Primary follicles | Secondary follicle | Mature follicle | Ovulation | Corpus luteum | Corpus albicans |

Oestrogens

Progesterone and oestrogens

Uterine cycle

Stratum functionalis

Stratum basalis

Days 0   7   **14**   21   28

Menstrual phase   Preovulatory phase   Ovulation   Postovulatory phase

Source: Peate I, Wild K & Nair M (eds). Nursing Practice: Knowledge and Care (2014).

Figure 42.2 Changes in the concentration of anterior pituitary and ovarian hormones.

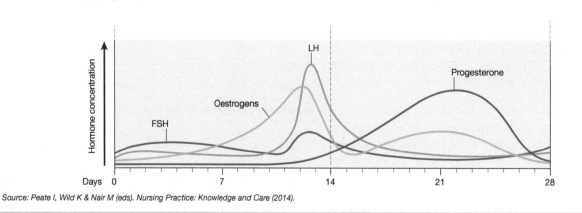

Source: Peate I, Wild K & Nair M (eds). Nursing Practice: Knowledge and Care (2014).

Anatomy and Physiology for Nursing and Healthcare Students at a Glance, Second Edition. Ian Peate.
© 2022 John Wiley & Sons Ltd. Published 2022 by John Wiley & Sons Ltd.
Companion website: www.wiley.com/go/peate/anatomyandphysiology

The reproductive cycle

The menstrual cycle is the series of changes a woman's body goes through to prepare for a pregnancy. The key participants in the female reproductive cycle are the pituitary gland, the ovaries and the uterus; the activities of each of these are very closely co-ordinated.

The reproductive cycle encompasses a series of events that occur regularly every 26–30 days throughout the child-bearing period. Each month, one of the ovaries releases a single egg (ovum). This is called ovulation and it occurs as a result of a complex set of interactions. There are three sets of hormones that control the menstrual cycle.

- Gonadotrophin-releasing hormones – luteinising hormone-releasing hormone (LHRH) and follicle-stimulating hormone-releasing hormone (FSHRH).
- Gonadotrophins – luteinising hormone (LH) and follicle-stimulating hormone (FSH).
- Ovarian hormones – oestrogen and progesterone.

Figure 42.1 provides an overview of the hormonal regulation of the changes in the ovary and uterus. Figure 42.2 describes the changes in the concentration of anterior pituitary and ovarian hormones.

The pituitary gland

The hypothalamus controls the actions of the pituitary gland; the menstrual cycle begins when the nerve cells in the hypothalamus trigger the secretion of FSH and LH. The gonadotrophin hormone-releasing factors from the hypothalamus control the release of the pituitary hormones (the gonadotrophins) – FSH and LH. They are produced by the anterior pituitary gland and they control the ovarian hormones oestrogen and progesterone.

The follicular phase

Also called the proliferative phase, this is considered the first phase of the menstrual cycle that leads to ovulation: it is when the ovary prepares to release an egg. The cycle usually lasts for 28 days and the follicular phase is the first 14 days of the cycle. During the follicular phase, there is a rise in FSH from the pituitary gland that stimulates the development of several follicles on the surface of the ovary; each follicle contains an egg. As the FSH level decreases, only one of the follicles continues to develop. This follicle also produces oestrogen. The endometrium prepares itself for the egg. In the early follicular phase, when menstrual flow has ended, the lining of the uterus is at its thinnest and levels of oestrogen and progesterone are at their lowest. Further on in the follicular phase, proliferation (or thickening) of the uterine lining occurs.

The ovulatory phase

Ovulation is the key event of the menstrual cycle. During each cycle, only one egg/ovule is released from the dominant ovarian follicle as it responds to a surge in LH and can only be fertilised for up to 48 hours.

This phase of the cycle occurs when there is a surge in pituitary LH secretion and concludes with the extrusion of the mature ovum through the capsule of the ovary.

The LH peaks mid-cycle; this then triggers the release of the ovum (ovulation), which usually happens 16–32 hours after the surge of LH begins. A couple of days later, the levels of LH fall. The oestrogen level from the ovaries increases gradually towards ovulation and peaks during the LH surge; this is key to ovulation.

The level of progesterone starts to rise towards follicle release, which prepares the endometrial lining of the uterus for implantation.

The luteal phase

During post ovulation, known as the luteal or premenstrual phase, the levels of LH and FSH decrease. After releasing the ovum, the ruptured follicle closes and forms a corpus luteum, which produces large amounts of progesterone. The progesterone prevents oestrogen from stimulating another surge of LH from the pituitary gland. If the ovum is fertilised, the progesterone levels are maintained by the corpus luteum and the endometrium is maintained.

If the egg is fertilised by sperm and then implants in (or attaches to) the endometrium, a pregnancy begins. This pregnancy is dated from day 1 of this menstrual cycle. If fertilisation does not occur, the corpus luteum starts to degenerate and progesterone and oestrogen levels begin to fall. The endometrial blood vessels constrict and the endometrial lining breaks down and is shed.

The menstrual cycle

The first day of the cycle is counted as the first day of the bleed – day 1. The cycle runs from the first day of menstruation to the next first day; 28 days is the average cycle length but the cycle can be shorter or longer. A teenager's cycle may be long (up to 45 days), becoming shorter over several years. Between 25 and 35 years, most women's cycles are regular and they generally last 21–35 days. At about 40–42 years, cycles tend to be the shortest and most regular. This is followed by 8–10 years of longer, less predictable cycles until the menopause occurs.

Menstruation is largely an endometrial event and is prompted by the loss of progesterone provided by the corpus luteum that occurs in non-conception cycles. In the endometrium, extraordinary structural changes occur during menstruation; some of these changes are understood but others are not.

> **Clinical practice point**
> Dysmenorrhoea is the term used to describe painful periods. Dysmenorrhoea is painful cramping, usually in the lower abdomen, which occurs shortly before or during menstruation, or both. Period pain from the woman's first period or shortly after and without a specific cause is known as primary dysmenorrhoea. Period pain caused by certain reproductive disorders, for example endometriosis, adenomyosis or fibroids, is known as secondary dysmenorrhoea.

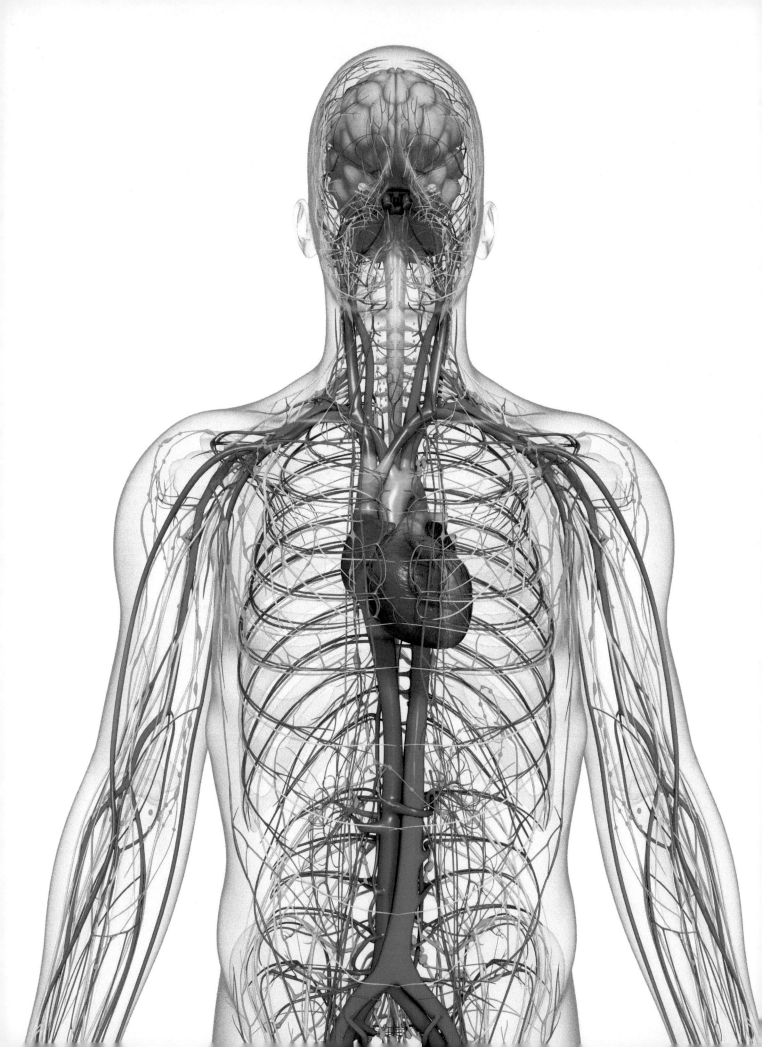

The endocrine system

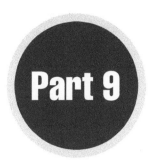

Part 9

43 The endocrine system

Figure 43.1   The major endocrine glands.

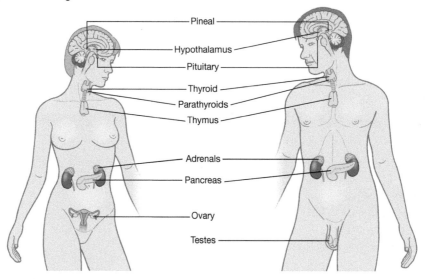

Pineal
Hypothalamus
Pituitary
Thyroid
Parathyroids
Thymus
Adrenals
Pancreas
Ovary
Testes

Figure 43.2   The pituitary gland and surrounding structures.

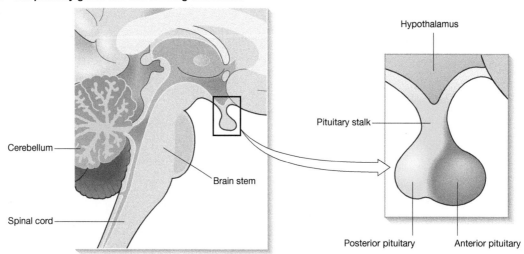

Hypothalamus
Pituitary stalk
Cerebellum
Brain stem
Spinal cord
Posterior pituitary   Anterior pituitary

Table 43.1 Hormones released by the hypothalamus and anterior pituitary gland.

Hypothalamus	Anterior pituitary gland	Target organ or tissues	Action
Growth hormone releasing factor (GHRF)	Growth hormone (GH)	Various (particularly bone)	Regulator of growth, metabolism and body structure
Growth hormone release inhibiting factor (GHRIF)	Growth hormone (inhibits release)	Various	
Thyroid releasing hormone (TRH)	Thyroid stimulating hormone (TSH)	Thyroid gland	Stimulates thyroid hormone release
Corticotrophin releasing hormones (CRH)	Adrenocorticotropic hormone (ACTH)	Adrenal cortex	Stimulates the release of corticosteroid
Prolactin releasing hormone (PRH)	Prolactin	Breasts	Stimulates the production of milk
Prolactin inhibiting hormone	Prolactin (inhibits release)	Breasts	
Gonadotropin releasing hormone (GRH)	Follicle stimulating hormone Luteinising hormone	Gonads	Numerous reproductive functions

Anatomy and Physiology for Nursing and Healthcare Students at a Glance, Second Edition. Ian Peate.
© 2022 John Wiley & Sons Ltd. Published 2022 by John Wiley & Sons Ltd.
Companion website: www.wiley.com/go/peate/anatomyandphysiology

There are 10 major endocrine glands (Figure 43.1).

The endocrine glands

The endocrine system is not as closely linked as other systems, for example the circulatory system. Endocrine glands are groups of secretory cells surrounded by a large network of capillaries; this rich blood supply permits diffusion of hormones (Table 43.1). In general, endocrine glands are ductless, vascular and most of them usually contain intracellular vacuoles or granules that store hormones. Exocrine glands, however, for example the salivary glands, mammary glands, sweat glands and those glands located within the gastrointestinal tract (for example, mucus glands), are usually much less vascular, with a duct or lumen to a membrane surface.

The pituitary gland and the hypothalamus

The hypothalamus is an aspect of the brain that has a number of functions; it is one of the most important parts of the nervous system. The pituitary gland is approximately 1 cm in diameter (the size of a pea) and is cone shaped (Figure 43.2). It rests in the hypophyseal fossa, a depression in the sphenoid bone under the hypothalamus. The gland is connected to the hypothalamus by a slender stalk called the infundibulum. The pituitary gland and the hypothalamus act as a unit, controlling most of the other endocrine glands.

Within the pituitary gland there are two distinct areas: the anterior lobe (adenohypophysis), composed of glandular epithelium, and the posterior lobe (neurohypophysis), made of a downgrowth of nervous tissue from the brain. Arterial blood supply is from the internal carotid artery with venous drainage (containing hormones) leaving the gland via short veins that enter the venous sinuses between the layers in the dura mater. The activity of the adenohypophysis is controlled by the release of hormones from the hypothalamus. The neurohypophysis is controlled by nerve stimulation.

The pineal gland

The pineal gland secretes the hormone melatonin which influences circadian rhythm (this is roughly a 24-hour cycle in the physiological processes of humans). The pinealocytes synthesise melatonin directly into the cerebrospinal fluid, which then takes it into the blood. Secretion of the hormone is controlled by daylight, with levels fluctuating throughout the day and seasons.

The anterior pituitary lobe

The anterior pituitary lobe (influenced by the hypothalamus) is supplied by arterial blood that has passed through the hypothalamus; blood is transported away from the gland via the pituitary portal system. The anterior pituitary lobe is larger than the posterior lobe and is formed of three parts; this partially surrounds the posterior lobe and infundibulum. This lobe is made up of glandular tissue producing and releasing hormones. There are no direct nerve connections with the anterior pituitary and the hypothalamus.

Control of the anterior pituitary occurs when releasing and inhibiting factors in the form of hormones are released by the hypothalamus.

Growth hormone (GH) stimulates the growth of bones, muscles and other organs by promoting protein synthesis. This hormone significantly affects the appearance of an individual as GH influences height.

Thyroid-stimulating hormone (TSH) causes the glandular cells of the thyroid to secrete thyroid hormone. If there is a hypersecretion of TSH, the thyroid gland enlarges, secreting excessive amounts of thyroid hormone.

Adrenocorticotrophic hormone (ACTH) reacts with receptor sites located in the cortex of the adrenal gland, stimulating the secretion of cortical hormones.

Gonadotrophic hormones react with receptor sites in the gonads, regulating the development, growth and function of the testes or ovaries.

Prolactin hormone encourages the development of glandular tissue in the female breast during pregnancy and stimulates the production of milk after the birth of the child.

The posterior pituitary lobe

The posterior pituitary is primarily composed of nerve fibres (a nerve bundle) that originate in the hypothalamus; the supporting nerve cells are called pituicytes. The hypothalamic–hypophyseal tract links the posterior pituitary and the hypothalamus (this is the nerve bundle). The posterior pituitary releases two hormones, which arrive directly from the hypothalamus:

- oxytocin
- antidiuretic hormone (ADH).

Oxytocin causes contraction of the smooth muscle in the wall of the uterus. It also stimulates the discharge of milk from the lactating breast; this is called the 'let-down' response and occurs in response to suckling when milk is released. The role of this hormone in males and non-lactating females is unclear; however, oxytocin is thought to play a role in sexual arousal and orgasm in men and women.

The key role of ADH (vasopressin) is to reduce urinary output. ADH promotes the reabsorption of water by acting on the distal convoluted tubules and collecting ducts of the nephrons of the kidneys, causing an increasing permeability to water. The result is that less water is lost as urine as reabsorption of water from the glomerular filtrate is increased. The amount of ADH that is secreted is controlled by the osmotic pressure of circulating blood to the osmoreceptors located in the hypothalamus. This mechanism conserves water for the body. Insufficient amounts of ADH cause excessive water loss in the urine. ADH secretion is stimulated by:

- increased plasma osmolality
- decreased extracellular volume
- pain and other stress conditions
- response to some drugs.

When there is a high concentration of ADH, for example after excessive blood loss or severe dehydration, smooth muscle contracts and vasoconstriction in small arteries occurs. This results in the pressor effect where systemic blood pressure is elevated.

Clinical practice point

Cushing disease occurs when the pituitary gland produces too much cortisol. The end result is overactive adrenal glands. Symptoms are varied and usually several are present which can include excessive and sudden (or at times more gradual) onset of weight gain around the trunk – arms and legs may remain unchanged and quite thin compared to the body; weak muscles, particularly in the legs; the face tends to be rounder and redder than usual (known as 'moon face'); acne may develop. Bones become weaker, due to steroid-induced osteoporosis. There may be hypertension, diabetes mellitus and a tendency to bruise easily with deep red/purple stretch marks (striae) on the abdomen. Some women experience irregular periods or stop having them. There may be excessive hair growth on parts of the body. Men can experience decreased fertility and in men and women there may be a disturbance in libido. There can be mood swings.

44 The thyroid and adrenal glands

Figure 44.1 The thyroid and parathyroid glands.

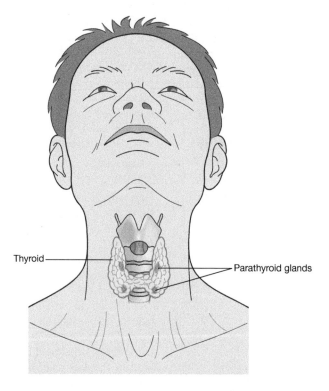

Thyroid

Parathyroid glands

Table 44.1 Some effects associated with abnormal secretion of thyroid hormones.

Increased secretion of T3 and T4 (hyperthyroidism)	Decreased secretion of T3 and T4 (hypothyroidism)
Increased basal metabolic rate	Decreased basal metabolic rate
Weight loss (despite good/increased appetite)	Weight gain (despite anorexia)
Tachycardia, palpitations, arrhythmia	Bradycardia
Excitability, nervousness, irritability	Tiredness, depression
Tremor	Numbness in the hands
Hair loss	Lifeless hair
Changes in menstruation patterns	Irregular menstrual periods
Goitre	Deep voice
Diarrhoea	Constipation
Exophthalmos	Feeling cold

Figure 44.2 Control of thyroid hormone production – negative feedback.

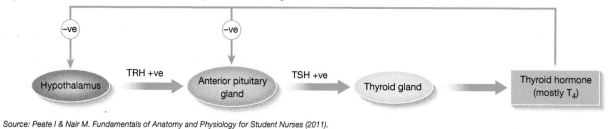

Source: Peate I & Nair M. Fundamentals of Anatomy and Physiology for Student Nurses (2011).

Anatomy and Physiology for Nursing and Healthcare Students at a Glance, Second Edition. Ian Peate.
© 2022 John Wiley & Sons Ltd. Published 2022 by John Wiley & Sons Ltd.
Companion website: www.wiley.com/go/peate/anatomyandphysiology

The thyroid gland

The thyroid gland is located in the neck, anterior to the larynx and the trachea, situated at the level of the 5th, 6th and 7th cervical vertebrae and the 1st thoracic vertebra. This is a butterfly-shaped gland (Figure 44.1) with two lobes located on either side of the thyroid cartilage and the upper incomplete cartilaginous rings of the trachea. It consists of a fibrous capsule weighing approximately 25 g, brownish red in colour. Lying in front of the trachea is the narrow isthmus joining the left and right lobes. Each lobe is cone shaped, measuring approximately 5 cm long and 3 cm wide.

The upper aspects of the lobes are known as the upper poles and lower ends the lower poles. The lobes are composed of hollow spherical follicles surrounded by capillaries.

The blood supply to this gland is extensive (it is said to be a highly vascular gland). The arterial blood supply comes from the superior and inferior thyroid arteries. Venous return is by the thyroid veins draining into the internal jugular vein. Principal innervation originates from the autonomic nervous system. Parasympathetic fibres come from the vagus nerves; sympathetic fibres are distributed from the superior, middle and inferior ganglia of the sympathetic trunk. These small nerves enter the gland accompanied by the blood vessels. Autonomic nervous regulation of the glandular secretion is not fully understood.

Lying against the posterior surfaces of each lobe are the parathyroid glands embedded in the thyroid tissues. The recurrent laryngeal nerve passes upwards and close to the lobes of the gland. A single layer of epithelial cells makes up the follicles, which form a cavity containing thyroglobulin molecules that are attached to iodine molecules; the thyroid hormones are formed by these molecules.

This gland releases two types of thyroid hormone: thyroxine (T4) and tri-iodothyronine (T3.) Iodine is essential for the synthesis of these hormones. Dietary iodine is concentrated by the thyroid gland and is changed into iodine in the follicle cells. Thyroid-stimulating hormone (TSH) stimulates thyroid hormone production.

The primary hormone released by the thyroid gland is T4, which is converted into T3 by the target cells. Thyroid hormones are required for normal growth and development. When there is deficiency of iodine, TSH is secreted in excess, causing proliferation of thyroid gland cells accompanied by an enlargement of the gland.

Table 44.1 outlines common effects associated with abnormal thyroid hormone secretion. Most of the cells in the body are affected by thyroid hormone, including an increase in basal metabolic rate and production of heat.

The regulation of thyroid hormone secretion is via a negative feedback mechanism involving the amount of circulating hormone, the hypothalamus and the adenohypophysis (Figure 44.2).

The parafollicular cells of the thyroid gland secrete calcitonin. Calcitonin combats the action of the parathyroid glands by reducing the levels of calcium in the blood. If blood calcium becomes too high, calcitonin is secreted until calcium ion levels decrease to normal.

Parathyroid glands

The four small masses of epithelial tissue embedded in the connective tissue capsule on the posterior surface of the thyroid glands are the parathyroid glands (see Figure 44.1). They are responsible for intestinal calcium absorption, stimulation of renal calcium absorption and stimulation of osteoclast activity and as such the reabsorption of calcium from the bones. Parathyroid hormone is secreted in response to low blood calcium levels and its effect is to increase those levels.

Hypoparathyroidism, or inadequate secretion of parathyroid hormone, leads to increased nerve excitability. The low blood calcium levels trigger spontaneous and continuous nerve impulses, which then stimulate muscle contraction. Calcium is also required for the creation of clotting factors in the blood which is monitored by cells in the gland. A reduction in blood calcium levels leads to an increase in the formation and secretion of parathyroid hormone.

The adrenal glands

The adrenal glands are located near the upper portion of each kidney. Each gland has an outer cortex and an inner medulla. The cortex and medulla, like the anterior and posterior lobes of the pituitary, secrete different hormones. The adrenal cortex is essential to life; the medulla may be removed with no life-threatening effects.

The hypothalamus influences both aspects of the adrenal gland but uses different mechanisms. The adrenal cortex is regulated by negative feedback involving the hypothalamus and adrenocorticotrophic hormone; the medulla is regulated by nerve impulses from the hypothalamus.

Hormones of the adrenal cortex

The adrenal cortex consists of three different regions; each region produces a different group or type of hormone. All the cortical hormones are steroid.

The outermost region of the adrenal cortex secretes mineralocorticoids; aldosterone is the chief mineralocorticoid, conserving sodium ions and water in the body. The middle region of the adrenal cortex secretes glucocorticoids. The key glucocorticoid is cortisol, increasing levels of blood glucose.

The third group of steroids is the gonadocorticoids (sex hormones), secreted by the innermost region. Male hormones (androgens) and female hormones (oestrogens) are secreted in minimal amounts in both sexes by the adrenal cortex; their effect is often masked by hormones from the testes and ovaries. In females, the masculinising effect of androgen secretion can become evident after menopause as levels of oestrogen from the ovaries decrease.

Hormones of the adrenal medulla

The adrenal medulla secretes two hormones, epinephrine and norepinephrine, in response to stimulation by sympathetic nerves, predominantly during stressful situations. A lack of hormones from the adrenal medulla will have no significant effects. Hypersecretion causes prolonged or continual sympathetic responses.

> **Clinical practice point**
>
> Hyperthyroidism is a condition where the thyroid gland produces more thyroid hormones than are needed by the body. It is also known as thyrotoxicosis or an overactive thyroid. It can occur if a person has Graves' disease, a toxic multinodular goitre, a solitary toxic thyroid adenoma (adenoma is a clump of cells) or thyroiditis (inflammation of the thyroid gland) which is temporary. Hypothyroidism is the condition resulting from an underactive thyroid gland. Hypothyroidism can be caused by autoimmune thyroid disease (Hashimoto thyroiditis), undergoing treatment for thyroid cancer or to correct hyperthyroidism, from specific medicines and an excessive intake of certain foods, a malfunction of the pituitary gland and radiation for head and neck cancers.

45 The pancreas and gonads

Figure 45.1 The pancreas.

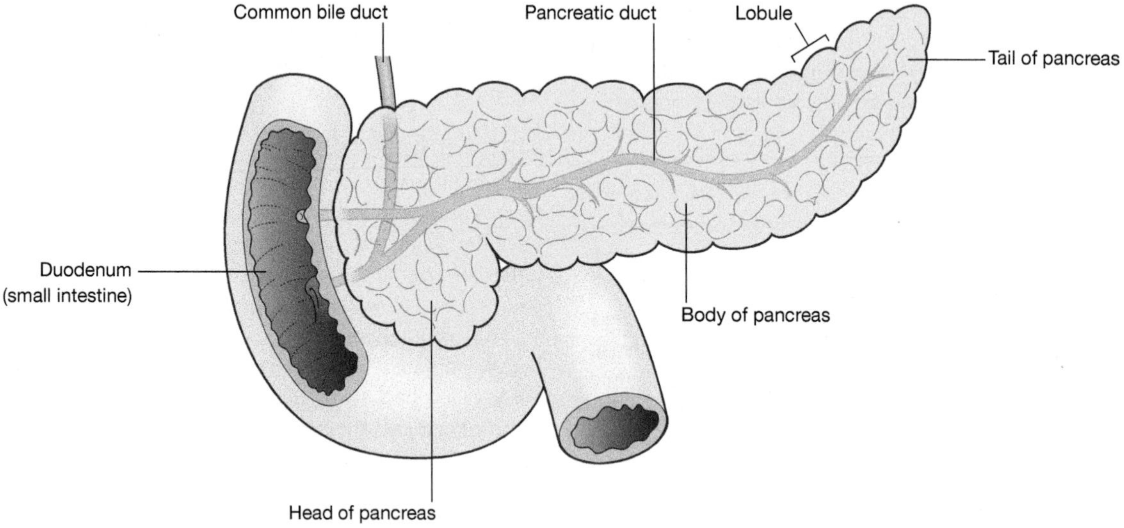

Common bile duct
Pancreatic duct
Lobule
Tail of pancreas
Duodenum (small intestine)
Body of pancreas
Head of pancreas

Figure 45.2 Insulin and glucagon effects on blood glucose.

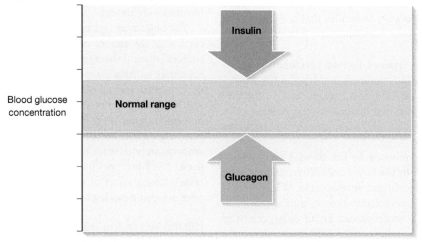

Blood glucose concentration

Insulin

Normal range

Glucagon

Source: Peate I & Nair M. Fundamentals of Anatomy and Physiology for Student Nurses (2011).

Table 45.1 Other endocrine glands.

Organ	Description
Thymus gland	Thymosin, a hormone produced by the thymus gland, has an important role in the development of the immune system
Stomach	The lining of the stomach, the gastric mucosa, produces gastrin, when food is present in the stomach. This stimulates the production of hydrochloric acid and the enzyme pepsin, used in the digestion of food
Small intestine	The mucosa of the small intestine secretes secretin and cholecystokinin when secreted promotes the pancreas to produce a fluid that neutralises the stomach acid. Cholecystokinin stimulates contraction of the gallbladder, releasing bile and stimulates the pancreas to secrete digestive enzyme
Heart	The heart also acts as an endocrine organ as well as pumping blood. Special cells in the wall of the atria produce atrial natriuretic hormone, or atriopeptin
Placenta	The placenta develops as a source of nourishment and gas exchange for the developing foetus. It also serves as a temporary endocrine gland. One hormone it secretes is human chorionic gonadotropin which signals the woman's ovaries to secrete hormones to maintain the uterine lining so that it does not degenerate and slough off in menstruation

Anatomy and Physiology for Nursing and Healthcare Students at a Glance, Second Edition. Ian Peate.
© 2022 John Wiley & Sons Ltd. Published 2022 by John Wiley & Sons Ltd.
Companion website: www.wiley.com/go/peate/anatomyandphysiology

The pancreas

The pancreas is a pale grey elongated gland (Figure 45.1), located in the epigastric and left hypochondriac regions of the abdomen. The head of the pancreas lies close to the first part of the small intestine – the duodenum – and the body behind the stomach, while the tail extends out towards to the spleen. It is about 12–15 cm in length and weighs approximately 60 g.

Blood supply to the pancreas comes from the splenic and mesenteric arteries. The splenic and mesenteric veins drain the pancreas where this drainage joins and forms the portal vein. The pancreas is innervated by the parasympathetic and sympathetic nervous systems. The secretion of insulin and glucagon is stimulated by the nervous system.

This gland has both endocrine and exocrine functions. Most of the tissue within the pancreas is made up of exocrine tissue and associated ducts.

The exocrine pancreas

The exocrine aspect of the gland is made up of a number of lobules that are composed of acini secreting digestive enzymes that are carried to the duodenum. The function of the exocrine element is to produce pancreatic juice that is rich in enzymes whose responsibility is to digest carbohydrates, protein and fats.

The endocrine pancreas

The endocrine portion is scattered throughout the exocrine tissue and consists of the pancreatic islets (the islets of Langerhans). The islets are the endocrine cells of the pancreas, which secrete insulin and glucagon. The islets have no ducts so the hormones are diffused directly into the blood. The islets have three key cell types, each producing a different hormone.

- Alpha cells secreting glucagon.
- Beta cells secreting insulin – these are the most abundant of the three cell types.
- Delta cells secreting somatostatin.

All three cell types are specifically placed within the islets' beta cells and are located in the central aspect of the islet surrounded by the alpha and delta cells. As the islets are highly vascularised, this enables the transportation of the hormones into the blood to occur at speed.

Insulin

This hormone is responsible for a number of things, including its effect on protein, mineral and lipid metabolism; one of its most well-known responsibilities is its ability to reduce blood glucose levels (Figure 45.2). Insulin facilitates the movement of glucose into muscle, adipose and other tissues (the brain and liver do not require insulin for the uptake of glucose). Insulin stimulates the liver to store glucose as glycogen.

Insulin synthesis is (principally) in response to a rise in blood glucose levels, and increases in blood, amino acids and fatty acids also have a stimulating effect. When blood glucose levels drop, there is a matching drop in insulin production and secretion, glycogen synthesis in the liver is reduced and enzymes responsible for the breakdown of glycogen are activated.

Glucagon

This hormone is also responsible for the maintenance of normal blood glucose. Glucagon has the opposite effects on blood glucose to insulin (see Figure 45.2). Glucagon increases blood glucose levels by stimulating the conversion of glycogen to glucose in the liver and skeletal muscles. Low blood sugar levels, exercise and decreased somatostatin and insulin stimulate the secretion of glucagon.

Somatostatin

Somatostatin inhibits the release of insulin and glycogen; when this hormone is released, it has effects locally. The exact functions of this hormone are unknown.

The gonads

The gonads are the primary reproductive organs: the testes in the male and the ovaries in the female. These organs are responsible for producing the sperm and ova and also secrete hormones and as such are considered endocrine glands.

The ovaries

Chapters 39 and 40 discuss the functions of the female reproductive system in detail.

The ovaries produce two groups of female sex hormones which are the oestrogens and progesterone. These are steroid hormones and contribute to the development and function of the female reproductive organs and sex characteristics. At the onset of puberty, oestrogens promote breast development, fat distribution and maturation of reproductive organs such as the uterus and vagina.

Progesterone causes the uterine lining to thicken in preparation for pregnancy. Progesterone and oestrogens are responsible for the changes occurring in the uterus during the female menstrual cycle.

The testes

Chapter 36 discusses the functions of the male reproductive system in detail.

Male sex hormones are called androgens. The main androgen is testosterone, secreted by the testes; the adrenal cortex also produces a small amount. Testosterone production starts during fetal development, continuing for a short time after birth, almost ceases during childhood and then resumes at puberty. This hormone is responsible for the growth and development of the male reproductive structures, increased skeletal and muscular growth, enlargement of the larynx accompanied by voice changes, growth and distribution of body hair and increased male sexual drive.

The secretion of testosterone is regulated by a negative feedback system involving the release of hormones from the hypothalamus and gonadotrophins from the anterior pituitary.

Other endocrine glands

In addition to the major endocrine glands discussed in this chapter, other organs have some hormonal activity as part of their function. Thesse include the thymus, stomach, small intestines, heart and placenta (Table 45.1).

Clinical practice point

Diabetes mellitus is a lifelong condition that causes a person's blood glucose level to become too high. There are two main types of diabetes. In type 1 diabetes the body's immune system attacks and destroys the cells that produce insulin. Type 2 diabetes arises when the body does not produce enough insulin, or the body's cells do not react to insulin. Gestational diabetes can occur during pregnancy; some women have such high levels of blood glucose that their body is unable to produce enough insulin to absorb it all. The amount of glucose in the blood is controlled by insulin, which is produced by the pancreas. When food is digested and enters the bloodstream, insulin moves glucose out of the blood and into cells, where this is broken down to produce energy. However, if the person has diabetes, their body is unable to break down glucose into energy. This is because there is either not enough insulin to move the glucose or the insulin that is produced does not work effectively. There are no lifestyle changes that can be made to lower the risk of type 1 diabetes. Lifestyle changes that can be instigated to reduce the risk of type 2 diabetes include healthy eating, regular exercise and achieving a healthy body weight.

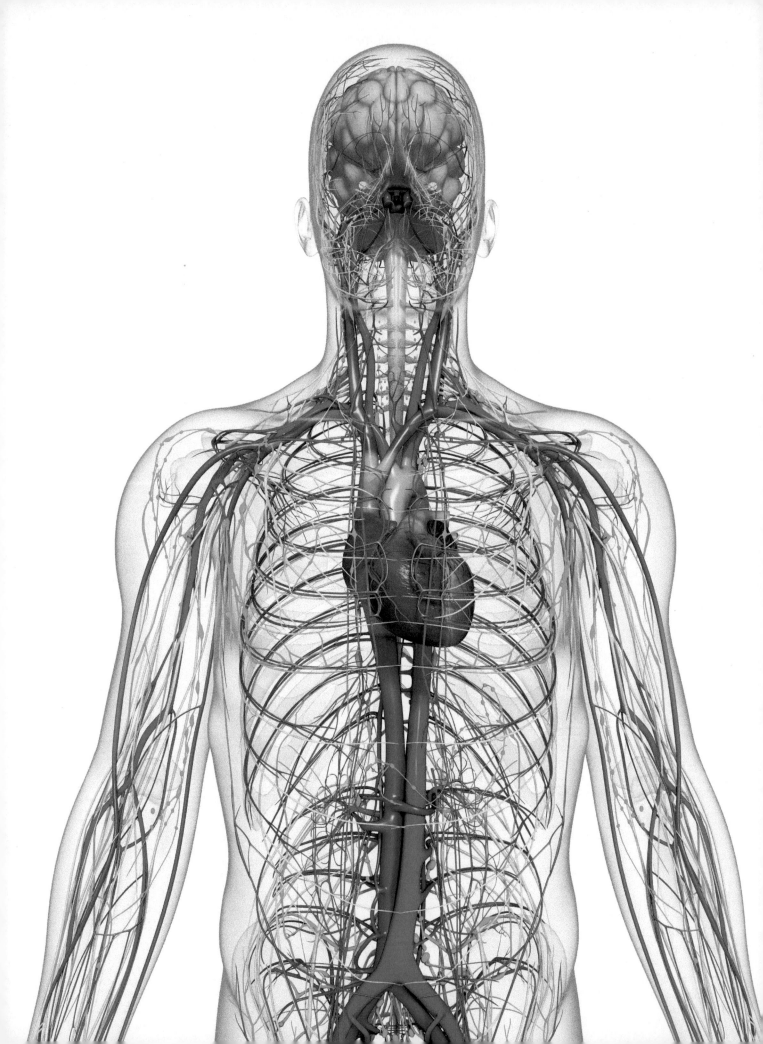

The musculoskeletal system

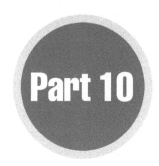

Part 10

Chapters

46 Bone structure

Figure 46.1 Bone remodelling.

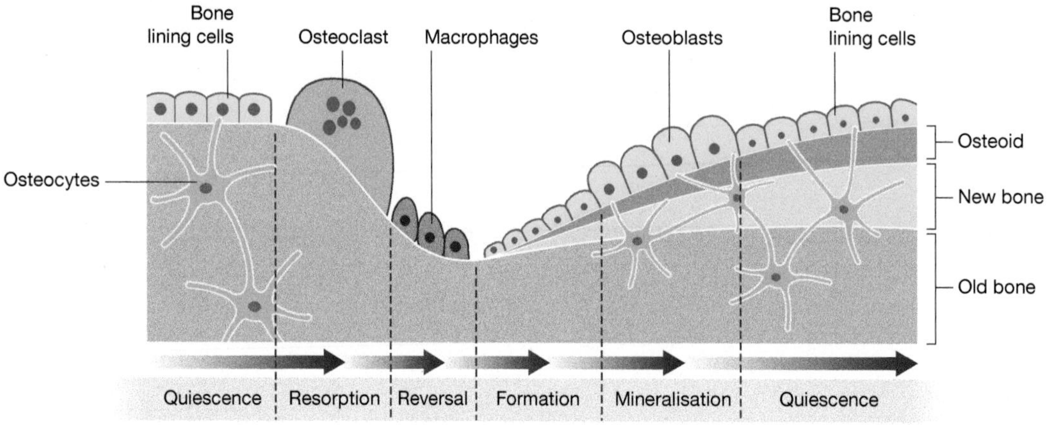

Bone
lining cells   Osteoclast   Macrophages   Osteoblasts   Bone
lining cells

Osteocytes

Osteoid
New bone
Old bone

Quiescence | Resorption | Reversal | Formation | Mineralisation | Quiescence

Source: Peate I, Wild K & Nair M (eds). Nursing Practice: Knowledge and Care (2014).

Figure 46.2 Bone growth.

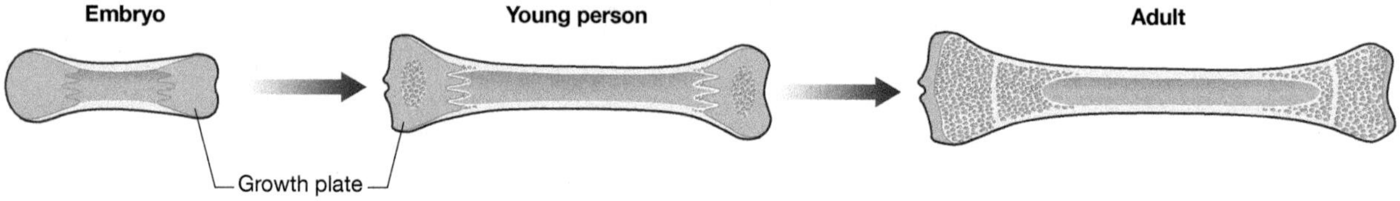

Embryo   Young person   Adult

Growth plate

Figure 46.3 Osteon, Haversian canal.

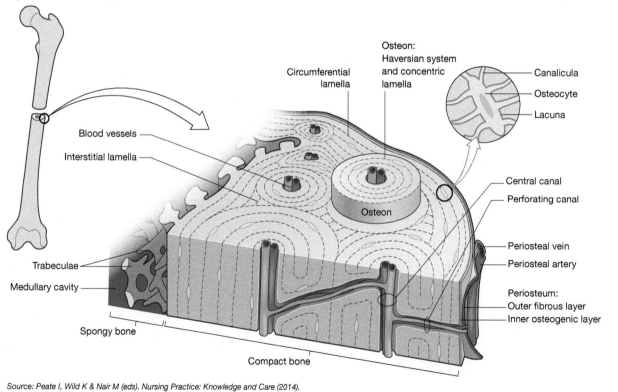

Circumferential
lamella

Osteon:
Haversian system
and concentric
lamella

Canalicula
Osteocyte
Lacuna

Blood vessels

Interstitial lamella

Osteon

Central canal

Perforating canal

Periosteal vein

Periosteal artery

Trabeculae

Medullary cavity

Periosteum:
Outer fibrous layer
Inner osteogenic layer

Spongy bone

Compact bone

Source: Peate I, Wild K & Nair M (eds). Nursing Practice: Knowledge and Care (2014).

Anatomy and Physiology for Nursing and Healthcare Students at a Glance, Second Edition. Ian Peate.
© 2022 John Wiley & Sons Ltd. Published 2022 by John Wiley & Sons Ltd.
Companion website: www.wiley.com/go/peate/anatomyandphysiology

Bone

Bone is living material, made up of minerals, consisting of living tissue and non-living substances. Bone is a dynamic tissue that continues to be built, broken down and rebuilt in a process called bone remodelling.

Bone structure can be compared to reinforced concrete used to make a building or a bridge. When the building or bridge is first assembled, an initial frame is put in place containing long steel rods. Cement is then poured around the rods. The rods and the cement form a close-fitting union, creating a structure that is strong and resilient enough to survive a rocking motion whilst also maintaining strength. If the steel rods were not present, then the cement would be brittle and liable to fracture even when only minor movements are made. Without the cement, the steel rods would have insufficient support, and would bend.

The same organisation is true of bone. The steel rods are the collagen rods in bone. The cement surrounding and supporting the rods is formed by minerals (calcium and phosphorus) from the blood that crystallise and surround the rods. Minerals provide the bones with strength and the collagen rods provide flexibility.

Bone remodelling and modelling

As we age, the skeleton changes. Throughout childhood, bone formation and growth occur with a gradual loss of bone density beginning in early adulthood and increasing significantly in older adults. During the process of ossification, calcium is used to create bone as the child grows and matures. Gradually, bone becomes hard and strong.

The density of bone is controlled by a group of cells including osteoclasts; these multinucleated cells resorb bone. Osteoblasts refill the cavities created by osteoclasts.

Bone resorption and formation is known as remodelling. Bone modelling occurs when there is an increase in bone mass. It promotes the growth of bones and is important for maintaining bone strength. Remodelling plays an important role in bone growth by improving the growing structure (Figure 46.1).

Those over 30 years of age usually experience a gradual loss in bone mass as there is a decrease in the activity of osteoblasts compared with osteoclasts. A number of factors play a part in the decrease in bone mass; for example, the use of glucocorticoids enhances the activity of the osteoclasts, reducing bone formation. Loss of bone mass reduces strength and increases the risk of fracture.

In the fetus, most of the skeleton is made up of cartilage, a tough, flexible connective tissue with no minerals or salts. As the fetus grows, osteoblasts and osteoclasts slowly replace cartilage cells and ossification begins (Figure 46.2).

Ossification

Ossification is the formation of bone by the activity of osteoblasts and osteoclasts and the addition of minerals and salts. Calcium compounds must be present for ossification to occur. Osteoblasts do not make these minerals, but take them from the blood and deposit them in bone. At birth, many of the bones have been at least partly ossified.

Within the bone are blood vessels, nerves, collagen and living cells, including osteoclasts and osteoblasts.

Osteoclasts

Bone tissue is continually broken down and resorbed by multinucleated cells called osteoclasts, derived from monocytes which originate in the bone marrow. Osteoclasts have an important role to play in freeing minerals and other molecules stored within the bone matrix.

Bone tissue serves as an important source of essential minerals, including calcium and phosphate, and other biological molecules such as growth factors. When calcium is released from the bone, this plays a role in maintaining homeostasis.

Osteoclasts are regulated by different signalling pathways and molecules. Increased osteoclast activity leads to increased resorption of bone.

Osteoblasts

These are the cells responsible for building new bone tissue. They are derived from cells thought to be associated with blood vessels. When activation occurs, they begin the production of the organic components of bone, including osteoid which is predominantly made of collagen. Minerals begin to crystallise around the collagen scaffold forming the major inorganic constituent of bone which contains calcium phosphate.

As osteoblasts form, new bone tissue may become embedded within the matrix, differentiating into osteocytes.

The structures and processes occurring within bone allow it to serve as a calcium reservoir whilst also providing structural support for the vital organs and movement.

The skeleton

The skeleton provides the body with shape and physical support for the systems contained within. The skeleton forms part of the musculoskeletal system which enables us to move.

The interior of bone is composed of bone marrow, surrounded by:

- cortical bone (the hard outer shell of bone)
- trabecular bone (the spongy centre).

The amount of cortical or trabecular tissue is dependent upon the function of the bone. The osteon is the basic unit of structure of compact bone, comprising a Haversian canal and its concentrically arranged lamellae (Figure 46.3).

Osteocytes are distributed within the lamellae, forming a network that maintains the viability and structural integrity of bone.

The Haversian canal is located at the centre of the osteon, containing blood vessels and nerves; blood vessels facilitate the exchange between the osteocytes and the blood. The vascular network provides structural support, nutrition and a waste removal system within this space.

Trabecular bone is present in the interior of some bones and resists compression; within the structure there are osteocytes, playing an important part in sensing local changes in strain.

In the interior of bones is the bone marrow. Bone marrow is a site for haematopoiesis, the process by which the cellular components of blood are formed.

Clinical practice point

Osteoporosis is a health condition that weakens bones, making them fragile and more likely to break (fracture). The most common injuries in people with osteoporosis are wrist, hip and vertebral (spinal) fractures. However, some fractures can also occur in other bones, for example the arm or pelvis. Fractured bones of the spine are a common cause of long-term pain. While a broken bone is often the first sign of osteoporosis, some older people will develop the characteristic stooped (bent forward) posture. Loss of bone is part of the ageing process, but some people lose bone much faster than normal. This can lead to osteoporosis and an increased risk of broken bones. Women also lose bone rapidly in the first few years following the menopause. Women are more at risk of osteoporosis than men, particularly if the menopause begins early (before the age of 45 years) or if their ovaries have been removed. Other factors can also increase the risk of developing osteoporosis: taking high-dose steroid tablets for longer than 3 months, other medical conditions, for example inflammatory conditions, hormone-related conditions or malabsorption problems, a family history of osteoporosis, long-term use of medicines that affect bone strength or hormone levels such as anti-oestrogen tablets, having or having had an eating disorder, having a low body mass index, not exercising regularly, heavy drinking and smoking.

47 Bone types

Figure 47.1 The skeleton: axial and appendicular.

Division of the skeleton	Structure	Number of bones	Division of the skeleton	Structure	Number of bones
Axial skeleton	• Skull		Appendicular skeleton	• Pectoral (shoulder) girdles	
	– Cranium	8		– Clavicle	2
	– Face	14		– Scapula	2
	• Hyoid	1		• Upper limbs	
	• Auditory ossicles	6		– Humerus	2
	• Vertebral column	26		– Ulna	2
	• Thorax			– Radius	2
	– Sternum	1		– Carpals	16
	– Ribs	24		– Metacarpals	10
	Number of bones	**80**		– Phalanges	28
				• Pelvic (hip) girdle	
				– Hip, pelvic, or coxal bone	2
				• Lower limbs	
				– Femur	2
				– Patella	2
				– Fibula	2
				– Tibia	2
				– Tarsals	14
				– Metatarsals	10
				– Phalanges	28
				Number of bones	**126**
				Total bones in an adult skeleton = 206	

Source: Peate I, Wild K & Nair M (eds). Nursing Practice: Knowledge and Care (2014).

Figure 47.2 Compact bone (long bone).

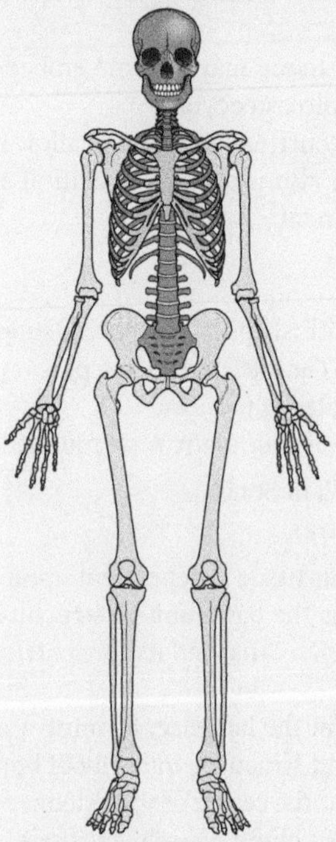

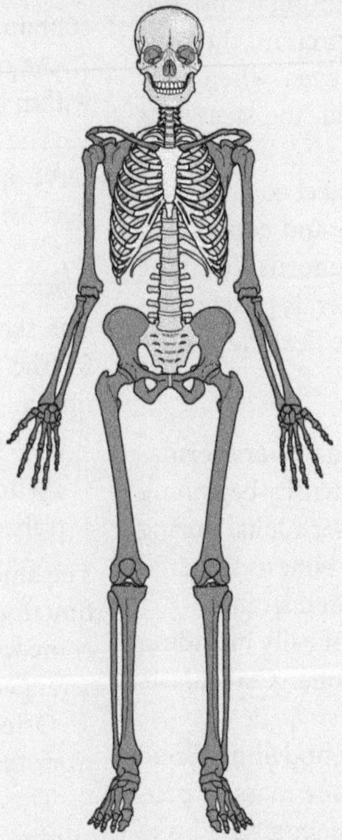

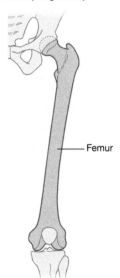

Femur

Figure 47.3 Short bone.

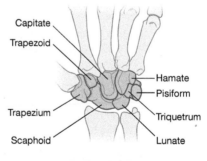

Capitate
Trapezoid
Hamate
Pisiform
Trapezium
Triquetrum
Scaphoid
Lunate

Figure 47.4 Flat bone.

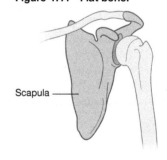

Scapula

Figure 47.5 Irregular bone.

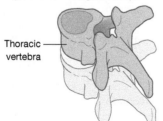

Thoracic vertebra

Figure 47.6 Sesamoid bone.

Patella

Anatomy and Physiology for Nursing and Healthcare Students at a Glance, Second Edition. Ian Peate.

Companion website: www.wiley.com/go/peate/anatomyandphysiology

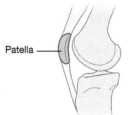

The skeleton

The human skeleton contains around 300 bones at birth but by the time the person reaches adulthood, this number has diminished to 206. As we age, smaller bones join together to make bigger bones – they fuse. The bones give the body its shape. The main job of the skeleton is to provide support for the body. Without the skeleton, the body would collapse into a heap. The skeleton is strong but light.

The skeleton also helps to protect the internal organs as well as the fragile body tissues. The skeleton protects the brain, eyes, heart, lungs and spinal cord. The cranium (skull) offers protection to the brain and eyes, while the ribs protect the heart and lungs and the vertebrae (spine, backbones) protect the spinal cord. Bones provide the structure for muscles to attach to so that we are able to move. Tendons are tough inelastic bands that attach muscle to bone. Red bone marrow makes blood cells and yellow marrow stores fat.

The study of bones is known as osteology.

Skeletal divisions

The bones make up the majority of the skeletal system and are divided into two groups: the axial skeletal bones and appendicular skeletal bones (Figure 47.1). In an adult human skeleton, there are 206 bones, 80 of which are from the axial skeleton and 126 from the appendicular skeleton.

The axial skeleton

The axial skeleton comprises the skull (includes bones of the cranium, face and ears [auditory ossicles]), the hyoid (U-shaped bone or complex of bones located in the neck between the chin and larynx), vertebral column (includes spinal vertebrae) and thoracic cage (includes ribs and sternum [breastbone]).

The appendicular skeleton

The appendicular skeleton is composed of body limbs and structures that attach limbs to the axial skeleton. Bones of the upper and lower limbs, pectoral girdle and pelvic girdle are elements of this aspect of the skeleton. Although the primary function of the appendicular skeleton is bodily movement, it also provides protection for organs of the digestive system, excretory system and reproductive system. The appendicular skeleton includes the pectoral girdle (includes shoulder bones [clavicle and scapula]), upper limbs (includes bones of the arms and hands), pelvic girdle (includes hip bones) and lower limbs (includes bones of the legs and feet).

Bone types

Bone types can be classified according to the shape and size of the bone. The shapes of bones reflect their functions. It is useful when describing specific bones to begin by stating the type of bone in relation to its shape; for example, the scapula is a large, flat, triangular bone. In terms of bone shape, there are five main types of bone:

- long bones
- short bones
- flat bones
- irregular bones
- sesamoid bones.

Bone tissue is classified as either compact bone or spongy bone and this depends on how the bone matrix and cells are organised. Compact bone forms the outer layer of all bones and most of the structure of long bones (Figure 47.2); it provides few spaces and offers protection and support as well as helping the long bones to bear the stress placed on them by body weight. Spongy bone (also called cancellous bone) has no osteons, but rather consists of an irregular lattice of thin columns of trabeculae. Spaces between the trabeculae of some spongy bones are filled with red bone marrow.

Long bones

These bones are often curved to assist with strength; they are longer and wider than other bones and consist of a shaft and a variable number of extremities (endings). The femur, tibia, fibula, humerus, ulna and radius are examples of long bones (see Figure 47.2).

Short bones

Short bones can be described as cube shaped and are approximately the same size lengthways and widthways. Their primary function is to provide support and stability with little movement. Examples of short bones are the carpals and tarsals – the wrist and foot bones. These consist of only a thin layer of compact, hard bone with cancellous bone on the inside with relatively large amounts of bone marrow (Figure 47.3).

Flat bones

Flat bones are strong, flat plates whose key function is to provide protection to the body's vital organs as well as being a base for muscular attachment. A prime example of a flat bone is the scapula (shoulder blade). The sternum (breastbone), cranium (skull), os coxae (hip bone), pelvis and ribs are also classed as flat bones. The anterior and posterior surfaces are formed of compact bone with the intention of providing strength for protection; the centre consists of cancellous (spongy) bone with varying amounts of bone marrow. The greatest number of red blood cells are formed in flat bones in adults (Figure 47.4).

Irregular bones

These bones do not fit into any other category, because of their non-uniform shape. Examples are the vertebrae, sacrum and mandible (lower jaw). They consist chiefly of cancellous bone, with a thin outer layer of compact bone (Figure 47.5).

Sesamoid bones

These types of bones are mostly short or irregular bones, embedded in a tendon. The patella (knee cap) is the most obvious example and sits within the patellar or quadriceps tendon. Other types of sesamoid bones are the pisiform (smallest of the carpals) and the two small bones at the base of the first metatarsal. Sesamoid bones are usually present in a tendon where it passes over a joint, which provides protection for the tendon (Figure 47.6).

> **Clinical practice point**
>
> Broken bones can happen after an accident such as a fall or by being hit by an object. The three most common signs of a fractured bone are pain, swelling and deformity. It can, however, be difficult to determine if a bone is fractured if it is not out of its normal position. With regard to breaking a bone, a snap or a grinding noise can be felt or heard as the injury happens, there may be swelling, bruising or tenderness around the injured area, pain may be felt when the person puts weight on the injury, touches it, presses it or moves it, the injured part may look deformed; in severe fractures, the bone may be appear through the skin. The person may also feel faint, dizzy or nauseous as a result of the shock. Medical help should be accessed as soon as possible if a broken bone is suspected.

Joints

Figure 48.1   Joint types.

Type of joint	Examples	Structure
Hinge	Elbow, knee 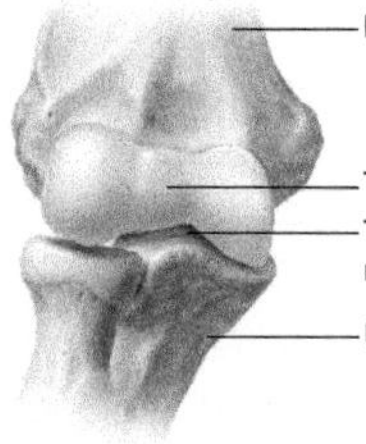 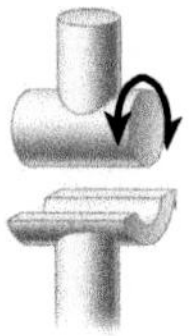	Humerus / Trochlea / Trochlear notch / Ulna
Pivot	Radius and ulna, the atlas and axis 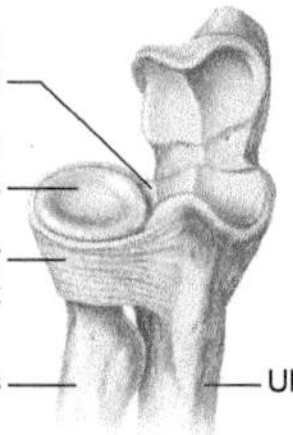 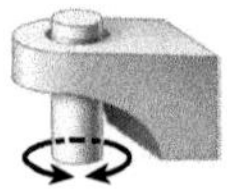	Radial notch / Head of radius / Annular ligament / Radius — Ulna
Ball and socket	Hip, shoulder 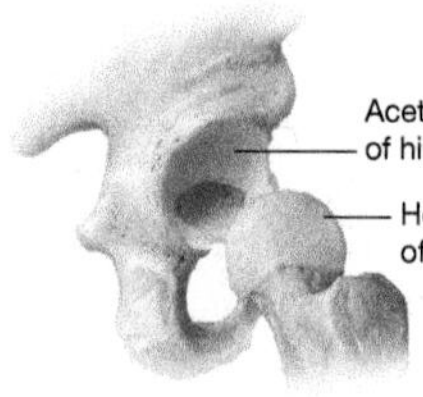 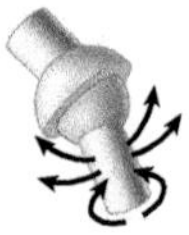	Acetabulum of hip bone / Head of femur
Saddle	The carpometacarpal joints of the thumb	Radius — Ulna / Trapezium / Metacarpal of thumb 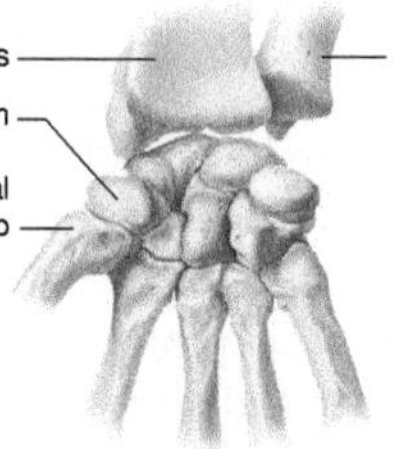 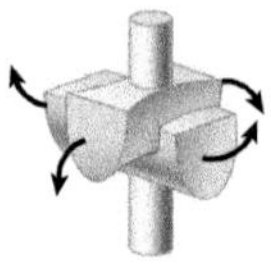
Condyloid	The radiocarpal and metacarpophalangeal joints of the hand 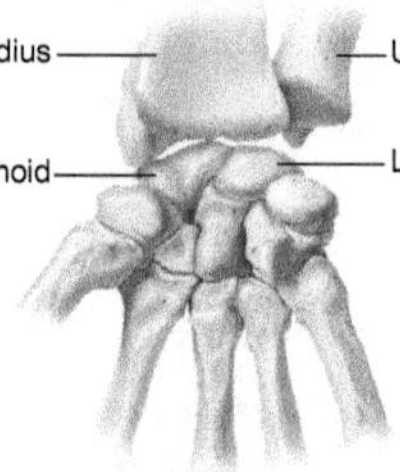 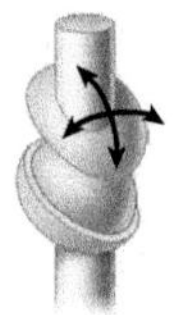	Radius — Ulna / Scaphoid — Lunate
Gliding	Intertarsal and intercarpal joints of the hands and feet 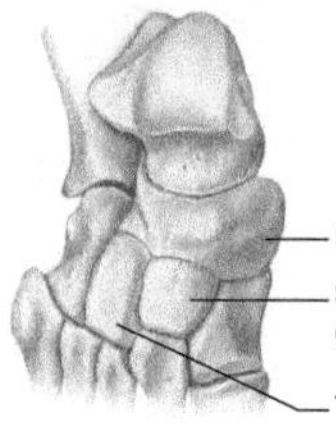 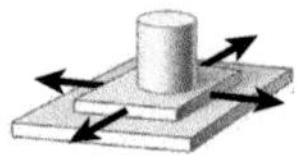	Navicular / Second cuneiform / Third cuneiform

Source: Peate I, Wild K & Nair M (eds). Nursing Practice: Knowledge and Care (2014).

Anatomy and Physiology for Nursing and Healthcare Students at a Glance, Second Edition. Ian Peate.
© 2022 John Wiley & Sons Ltd. Published 2022 by John Wiley & Sons Ltd.
Companion website: www.wiley.com/go/peate/anatomyandphysiology

Joints

Joints occur where two bones meet. All bone (apart from the hyoid bone in the neck) form a joint with another bone. Joints hold the bones together, joints are also called articulations.

Movements

The bones act as levers providing transmission of muscular forces. A number of bones can, through leverage, contracting and pulling, change the extent and direction of the forces generated by skeletal muscles, through the work of the tendons and the ligaments. These movements can be very intricate, such as the ability to write or thread a needle (co-ordination of fine movement), or more general (gross movement), such as the ability to move body position. The interaction of the skeleton with the muscles enables breathing to occur.

A tendon is a fibrous connective tissue attaching muscle to bone. Tendons can also attach muscles to structures such as the eyeball. A tendon helps to move the bone or structure. A ligament is a fibrous connective tissue attaching bone to bone, and generally serves to hold structures together, keeping them stable.

There are a number of different types of movement available at different joints; the shoulder joint, for example, moves in many more ways than the knee. These are the main types of movement.

- *Flexion*: reducing the angle at the joint, bending the knee or elbow.
- *Extension*: increasing the angle at the joint, for example straightening the knee or elbow.
- *Adduction*: moving the body part towards the centre of the body, for example bringing one leg in towards the other.
- *Abduction*: moving the body part away from the centre of the body, for example taking one leg away from the other.
- *Rotation*: turning or twisting a body part, either clockwise (external or lateral) or anticlockwise (internal or medial), for example turning the leg to point the toes outwards.

Fibrous joints

These are also called synarthrodial joints. They are held together by only a ligament. A ligament is dense irregular tissue that is made up of rich collagen fibres. There is no synovial cavity in this type of joint.

Cartilaginous joints

Cartilaginous joints are also known as synchondroses (singular synchondrosis) and symphyses (singular symphysis). They occur where the connection between the articulating bones is made up of cartilage with no synovial cavity, for example the joints between vertebrae in the spine.

Symphysis joints are permanent cartilaginous joints that have an intervening pad of fibrocartilage, for example the symphysis pubis.

Synovial joints

Also called diarthrosis joints, the most common classification of joint. They are extremely moveable, with an articular capsule enclosesing the whole joint, a synovial membrane (the inner layer of the capsule) which produces synovial fluid and hyaline cartilage padding the ends of the articulating bones.

Synovial fluid is a thin film that is usually viscous, clear or yellowish. It helps in preventing friction by providing the joint with lubrication, supplying nutrients and removing waste products.

There are six types of freely moveable, or synovial, joints (Figure 48.1).

The majority of joints are synovial joints which allow for much more movement than the cartilaginous joints. Synovial joints are mainly located in the limbs where mobility is essential. Ligaments help provide their stability and the muscles contract in order to produce movement.

Hinge

A convex portion of one bone fits into a concave portion of another bone. The movement reflects the hinge and bracket movement of a household hinge and bracket; movement is limited to flexion and extension. The joint produces an open and closing motion. These joints are uniaxial.

Pivot

A rounded part of one bone fits into the groove of another bone. These joints will only permit movement of one bone around another and are classified as uniaxial movement.

Ball and socket

The spherical end of one bone fits into a concave socket of another bone. Movement happens through flexion, extension and adduction. This is a triaxial joint.

Condyloid

Where an oval surface of one bone fits into a concavity of another bone and where condyloid joints are found. Permits flexion, extension and adduction. This is a biaxial joint.

Saddle

Similar to condyloid joints, but these joints permit greater movement. Allows flexion, extension and adduction. The joint is classed as triaxial.

Gliding

These joints have a flat or slightly curved surface enabling gliding movements. The joints are bound by ligaments and movement in all directions is restricted. The joint moves back and forth and from side to side.

Fixed joints

There are some joints, such as those in the skull, that are fixed and do not permit any movement to occur. The bones in the skull, for example, are held together with fibrous tissue, as are the joints in the pelvis.

Clinical practice point

Arthritis (inflammation of a joint) causes pain and inflammation in a joint. Arthritis affects people of all ages, including children. The two most common types of arthritis are osteoarthritis and rheumatoid arthritis. Osteoarthritis, the most common type of arthritis in the UK, often develops in people in their mid-40s or older. The condition is also more common in women and those with a family history of the condition. It can occur at any age as a result of an injury or be associated with other joint-related conditions, for example gout or rheumatoid arthritis. Osteoarthritis primarily affects the smooth cartilage lining of the joint, making movement more difficult than usual, leading to pain and stiffness.

49 Muscles

Figure 49.1   Muscle tissues.

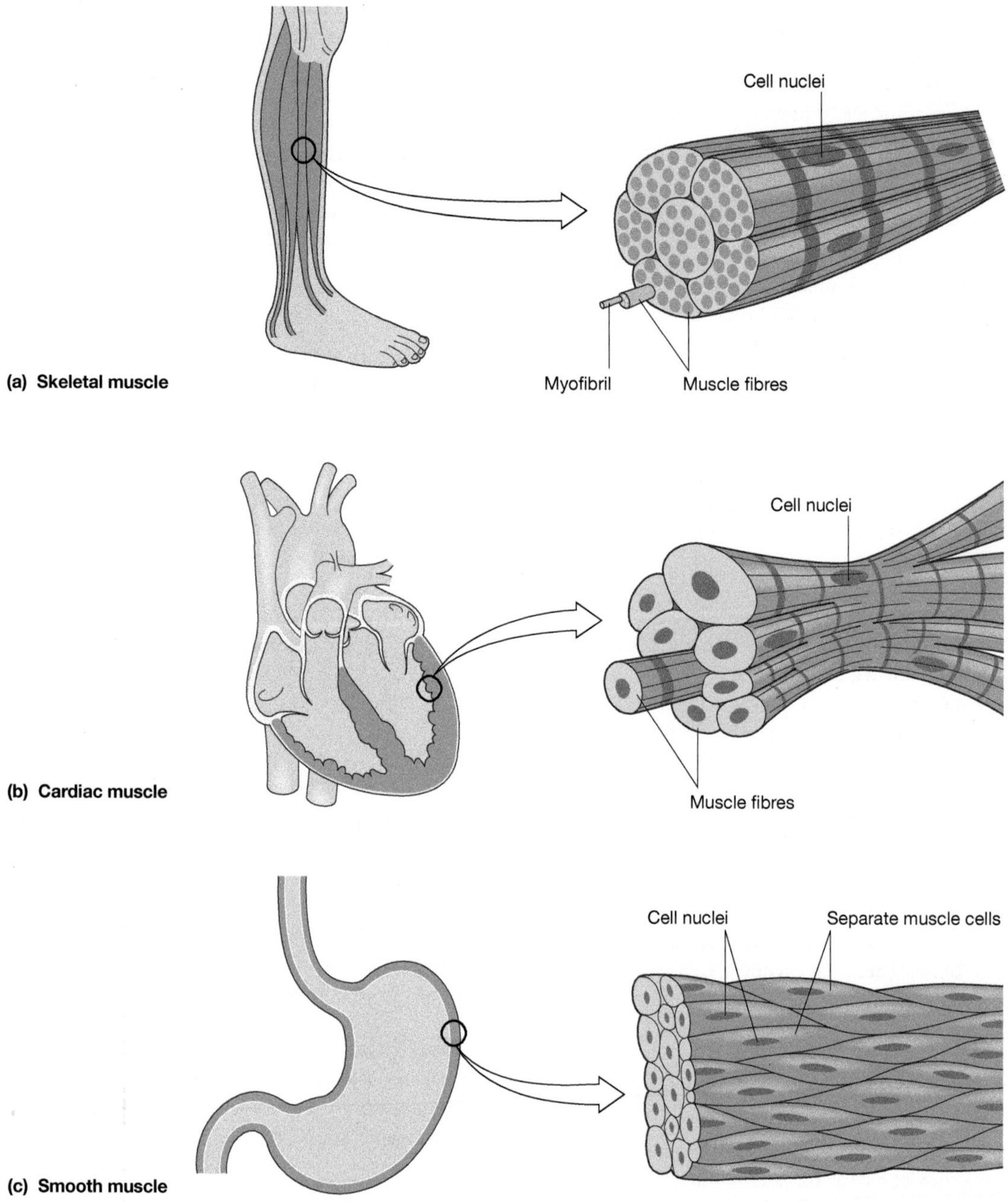

(a) Skeletal muscle

Cell nuclei

Myofibril   Muscle fibres

(b) Cardiac muscle

Cell nuclei

Muscle fibres

(c) Smooth muscle

Cell nuclei   Separate muscle cells

Anatomy and Physiology for Nursing and Healthcare Students at a Glance, Second Edition. Ian Peate.
© 2022 John Wiley & Sons Ltd. Published 2022 by John Wiley & Sons Ltd.
Companion website: www.wiley.com/go/peate/anatomyandphysiology

The bones provide the framework for the body as well as providing leverage but it is the muscles that pull the bones; muscles can only pull, they cannot push, and the bones cannot move body parts. Muscles contract and move the viscera and the blood vessels; cardiac muscle makes the heart beat. Energy is turned into locomotion by the muscles, helping to drive the body. Without muscles, we would not be able to do anything; each time we move, blink, swallow food, inhale and exhale, smile or frown, muscle is involved. Muscle tissue generates heat as it contracts. Much of this chapter will concentrate on skeletal muscle.

Muscle tissue

There are three types of muscle tissue: skeletal, cardiac and smooth (Figure 49.1).

Skeletal muscle tissue

This is made up of long single striated fibres. The fibres vary in length from a few centimetres to 40 cm and have many nuclei. This muscle is voluntary – it can be made to relax or contract as a result of conscious effort.

Skeletal muscle tissue is, as the name suggests, found in the skeletal muscles. The function of the majority of skeletal muscles is to move the bones. The function of skeletal muscle is to produce movement, maintain posture, produce heat and act in a protective manner.

Skeletal muscles are surrounded by connective tissue with a good nerve and blood supply. The individual cells (fibres) are ordinarily long and thin, but become shorter and fatter under stimulus and have the ability to sustain a tremendous pulling power. When the stimulus has passed, the muscle relaxes and returns to its original shape.

The sarcolemma is the muscle cell, the cytoplasm is the sarcoplasm. The tubules begin at the sarcolemma, extending into the sarcoplasm and permitting rapid distribution to contract throughout the muscle fibre. Muscle fibre contains myofibrils which are responsible for contraction. They consist of bundles of filaments made up of actin and myosin and are organised into functional units called sarcomeres. Actin filaments are thick and lie at the centre of the sarcomere, while myosin is made up of thin filaments at either end. The Z line separates the sarcomere and the M line is in the middle. Actin and myosin filaments are joined by cross-bridges, which engage and re-engage during contraction, resulting in shortening. Calcium is released by a number of structures promoting muscle contraction. Each fibre is surrounded by a layer of endomysium joined in bundles forming fascicles, each of which is covered in perimysium.

The structure that permits the nerve impulse to initiate contraction is called the neuromuscular junction (NMJ). Each muscle fibre has one NMJ where the axon of the neuron joins the fibre. At the terminal end of the axon, closest to the motor endplate, the nerve and motor endplate (not in direct contact) are separated by the synaptic cleft. The muscle is activated as a result of chemical transmission; the transmitter is acetylcholine contained in the axon which bonds to receptors located on the motor endplate.

Depolarisation of the sarcolemma occurs and the action potential spreads across the sarcolemma down the transverse tubules into the interior of the cells of the triads. Calcium is then released and the muscle contracts.

Cardiac muscle tissue

These are branched striated fibres; usually this type of muscle has only one centrally located nucleus. Each end is attached by transverse thickenings of plasma membrane containing desmosomes and gap junctions. The desmosomes bolster tissue and hold fibres together as forceful contraction occurs. The gap junctions allow for rapid conduction of electrical signals in the heart. This type of muscle is involuntary; the contractions are not consciously controlled.

This muscle is found only in the walls of the heart. Cardiac muscle functions in order to pump blood throughout the body.

Smooth muscle tissue

This is made of non-striated involuntary fibres and contains a single, centrally based nucleus. Gap junctions are present connecting many individual fibres; this permits powerful contractions of many muscle fibres in a unified manner, for example in the iris of the eye, the walls of hollow organs, the blood vessels, stomach, intestines, urinary bladder and uterus. Smooth muscle fibres contract separately as is the case with skeletal muscle.

Smooth muscle tissue provides wave-like movement such as occurs with the propulsion of food as it travels through the gastrointestinal tract, contraction of the stomach and the urinary bladder.

Properties of muscle tissue

There are four properties of muscle tissue.

- *Excitability* (irritability): ability to receive and respond to stimuli via the generation of an electrical pulse which results in contraction of the muscle cells.
- *Contractility*: ability to shorten.
- *Extensibility*: ability to be stretched or extended.
- *Elasticity*: ability of a muscle fibre to recoil and resume its resting length.

Clinical practice point

Myopathies are neuromuscular diseases which cause muscle fibres to lose function, resulting in muscle weakness. Congenital myopathy refers to a group of muscle disorders that appear at birth or in infancy; there are a number of types of congenital myopathy. Usually, an infant with a congenital myopathy will be 'floppy' (hypotonia), have difficulty breathing or feeding and may not meet their normal developmental milestones such as turning over or sitting up.

Muscle weakness can occur for a number of reasons, including a problem with the muscle, a problem with the nerve that stimulates the muscle or a problem with the brain. In order to diagnose a congenital myopathy, a neurologist will carry out a detailed physical examination as well as a range of tests to determine the cause of weakness. If a myopathy is suspected, potential tests will include a blood test for a muscle enzyme called creatine kinase, an electromyogram to evaluate the electrical activity of the muscle, a muscle biopsy and genetic testing.

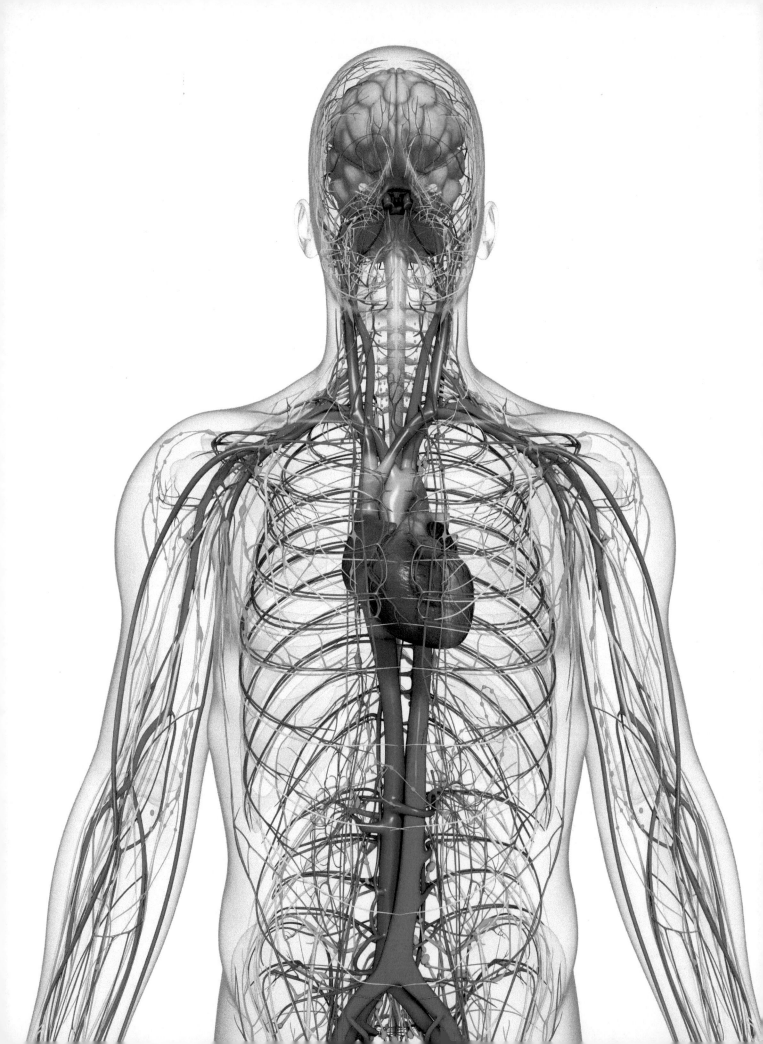

The skin

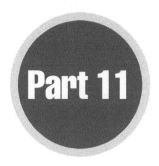
Part 11

Chapters

50 The skin

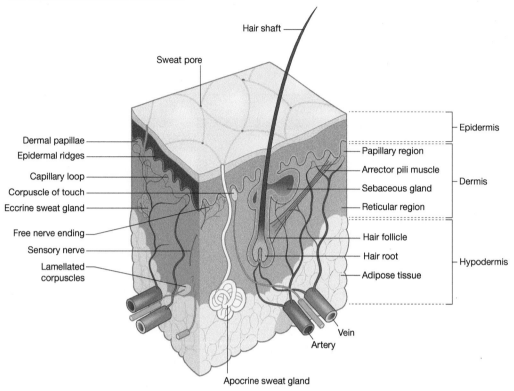

Figure 50.1   The skin and associated structures.

- Hair shaft
- Sweat pore
- Dermal papillae
- Epidermal ridges
- Capillary loop
- Corpuscle of touch
- Eccrine sweat gland
- Free nerve ending
- Sensory nerve
- Lamellated corpuscles
- Epidermis
- Papillary region
- Arrector pili muscle
- Sebaceous gland
- Reticular region
- Dermis
- Hair follicle
- Hair root
- Adipose tissue
- Hypodermis
- Vein
- Artery
- Apocrine sweat gland

Source: Peate I, Wild K & Nair M (eds). Nursing Practice: Knowledge and Care (2014).

Figure 50.2   Skin types.

	Natural skin colour	UV sensitivity and tendency to burn
1	Very fair, pale white, often freckled	**Highly sensitive** Always burns, never tans
2	Fair, white skin	**Very sensitive** Burns easily, tans minimally
3	Light brown	**Sensitive** Burns moderately, usually tans
4	Moderate brown	**Less sensitive** Burns minimally tans well
5	Dark brown	**Minimally sensitive** Rarely burns
6	Deeply pigmented, dark brown to black	**Minimal sensitivity** Never burns

Figure 50.3   The layers of the epidermis.

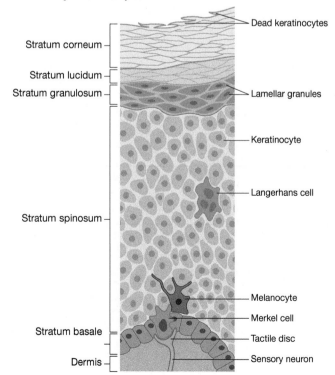

- Stratum corneum
- Stratum lucidum
- Stratum granulosum
- Stratum spinosum
- Stratum basale
- Dermis
- Dead keratinocytes
- Lamellar granules
- Keratinocyte
- Langerhans cell
- Melanocyte
- Merkel cell
- Tactile disc
- Sensory neuron

Anatomy and Physiology for Nursing and Healthcare Students at a Glance, Second Edition. Ian Peate.
© 2022 John Wiley & Sons Ltd. Published 2022 by John Wiley & Sons Ltd.
Companion website: www.wiley.com/go/peate/anatomyandphysiology

The skin (also known as the integumentary system) is the largest organ of the body. It accounts for approximately 15% of the total adult body weight and is composed of specialist cells and structures. The skin carries out a number of essential functions; these include protecting the person against external physical, chemical and biological attack, preventing the loss of excess water from the body and playing a key role in thermoregulation. The skin is continuous with the mucous membranes that line the surface of the body.

The skin and its derivatives, for example the hair, nails, sweat and oil glands, make up the integumentary system (see chapter 51). It is composed of three layers:

- the epidermis
- the dermis
- subcutaneous tissue (hypodermis). See Figure 50.1.

Throughout the body, the skin's characteristics vary; for instance, the head contains more hair follicles than anywhere else, while the soles of the feet contain none. The thickness of the layers of the skin varies depending on where it is located on the body. The eyelids have the thinnest layer of the epidermis, measuring less than 0.1 mm, while the palms of the hands and soles of the feet have the thickest epidermal layer, measuring approximately 1.5 mm. On the back the dermis is at its thickest, around 30–40 times thicker than the overlying epidermis. Skin type is another important characteristic (Figure 50.2). The skin is constantly renewed.

There are four types of tissues in the skin: the epidermis covers the surface of the body; connective tissue, made of protein fibres, is tough and flexible; muscle in the skin interacts with hairs responding to various stimuli including heat and fright; and nervous tissue enables us to detect external stimuli such as pain and pressure.

The layers of the skin

The epidermis

The epidermis is the thinner and more superficial layer of the skin, made up of four types of cell: keratinocytes, melanocytes, Langerhans cells and Merkel cells. The keratinocytes are the most common type of skin cells; they produce keratin which is a fibrous protein that helps protect the epidermis. Keratin provides strength to skin, hair and nails. Keratinocytes are formed in the deep, basal cell layer of the skin, gradually migrating upwards, where they become squamous cells prior to reaching the surface of the skin over the course of about 4 weeks. Melanocytes are responsible for synthesising the brown pigment melanin. Pigmentation is extremely heritable, regulated by genetic, environmental and endocrine factors that affect the amount, type and distribution of melanin in the skin, hair and eyes. Melanocytes are located in the lower part of the epidermis, just above the dermis. It is melanin that gives colour to the skin, hair and parts of the eye. Melanin also plays an important role in protecting the skin from the harmful radiation produced by ultraviolet (UV) light; it is an important defence system of the skin against harmful factors.

Langerhans cells are associated with immune response; they regulate immune reactions in the skin. These cells work by ingesting antigens that get into the skin, presenting them to cells of the immune system. The dendritic Langerhans cells originate in the bone marrow. They then migrate to the epidermis where they form a regularly arranged network that can reach a density of approximately 700–800 cells per square millimetre.

The touch receptor cells – the Merkel cells – participate in the sense of touch and are located primarily in the basal layer of the epidermis. There is much variation in the density of the Merkel cells; the fingertips and plantar aspects of the toes have a far greater density than any other part of the body.

There are five separate sublayers of the epidermis.

- *Stratum corneum*: the outermost layer has 25–30 layers of flat dead keratinocytes. Lamellar granules provide water-repellent action and are continuously shed and replaced.
- *Stratum lucidum*: this is only found in the fingertips, palms of hands and soles of feet. This layer is made up of 3–5 layers of flat dead keratinocytes.
- *Stratum granulosum*: made up of 3–5 layers of keratinocytes and is the site of keratin formation; keratohyalin gives it its granular appearance.
- *Stratum spinosum*: appears as if covered in thorn-like spikes, providing the skin with strength and flexibility.
- *Stratum basale*: this is the deepest layer, made up of a single layer of cuboidal or columnar cells. Cells produced in this layer are constantly dividing and move up to the surface (Figure 50.3).

The dermis

This layer is composed of connective tissue; blood vessels, nerves, glands and hair follicles, collagen and elastic fibres help with strength and elasticity. The normal cells in the dermis include mast cells, containing granules packed with histamine and other chemicals, released when the cell is disturbed; vascular smooth muscle cells that allow blood vessels to contract and dilate, required to control body temperature; specialised muscle cells such as myoepithelial cells found around sweat glands which contract to expel sweat. Fibroblasts produce and deposit collagen and other elements of the dermis as required for growth or to repair wounds.

There are many types of immune cell. The role of tissue macrophages (histiocytes) is to remove and digest foreign or degraded material (known as phagocytosis). There are also small numbers of lymphocytes in the normal dermis.

The functions of the adipocytes include sensitivity to insulin and the ability to produce and secrete adipocyte-specific endocrine hormones regulating energy homeostasis in other tissues; they are critical regulators of whole-body metabolism. Macrophages and fibroblasts play a central role in wound healing.

The two main divisions of the dermal layer are the papillary region in the superficial layer of the dermis, made up of loose areolar connective tissue with elastic fibres, and the dermal papillae which are finger-like structures invading the epidermis containing capillaries or Meissner corpuscles which respond to touch.

The subcutaneous tissues

Sometimes called the subcutis or hypodermis, this is the deepest layer of the skin.

Subcutaneous tissue is an important line of defence, composed of an insulating layer of fat and blood vessels. The size of this layer varies throughout the body and from person to person. The fat in the subcutaneous layer offers protection to the organs and bones, helping to maintain body temperature, working with the blood vessels to keep temperature normal and consistent. The sweat glands in this layer are also important in thermoregulation. As the body ages, subcutaneous tissue begins to thin out.

Clinical practice point

People with skin diseases may experience a significant negative psychosocial impact and reduced quality of life. Given the highly visible nature of dermatological conditions, stigmatisation is a common problem requiring significant consideration in those with skin diseases. Those with visible skin diseases can experience not only physical symptoms but also psychosocial consequences, for example depression, anxiety, impaired quality of life and low self-esteem.

51 The skin appendages

Figure 51.1 The hair and associated glands.

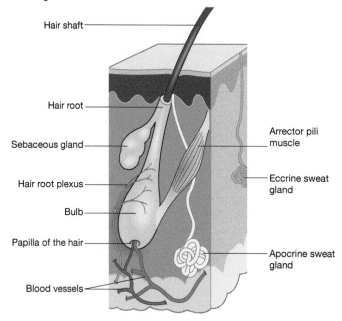

- Hair shaft
- Hair root
- Sebaceous gland
- Hair root plexus
- Bulb
- Papilla of the hair
- Blood vessels
- Arrector pili muscle
- Eccrine sweat gland
- Apocrine sweat gland

Source: Peate I, Wild K & Nair M (eds). Nursing Practice: Knowledge and Care (2014).

Figure 51.2 The nails.

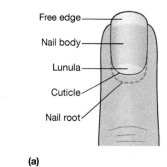

- Free edge
- Nail body
- Lunula
- Cuticle
- Nail root

(a)

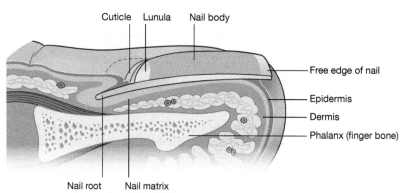

- Cuticle
- Lunula
- Nail body
- Free edge of nail
- Epidermis
- Dermis
- Phalanx (finger bone)
- Nail root
- Nail matrix

(b)

Source: Peate I, Wild K & Nair M (eds). Nursing Practice: Knowledge and Care (2014).

Anatomy and Physiology for Nursing and Healthcare Students at a Glance, Second Edition. Ian Peate.
© 2022 John Wiley & Sons Ltd. Published 2022 by John Wiley & Sons Ltd.
Companion website: www.wiley.com/go/peate/anatomyandphysiology

The appendages of the skin are sometimes also referred to as the derivatives of the integument. The appendages include the hair, the nails and the glands.

The dermal appendages

The hair

The hair provides a variety of functions including protection, thermoregulation and sensing light touch. Hair is composed of a variety of columns of dead, elongated keratinised cells bound together by extracellular proteins. There are two main parts of the hair.

- *The shaft*: this is the superficial portion that extends out of the skin.
- *The root*: this portion penetrates into the dermis.

The hair follicle is a small blind-ended tubular structure consisting of five concentric layers of epithelial cells extending from the dermis through to the epidermis containing the hair root. At the base of the hair follicle is a bulbous expansion, an onion-shaped structure (a bulb) that is called the papilla of the hair and the matrix contained within the bulb produces new hair. The sebaceous and the apocrine skin glands have ducts that lead into the hair follicle.

During hair formation, the inner three layers undergo keratinisation and the outer two layers form an epithelial sheath. At age 3 months, hairs begin to appear over the eyebrow and upper lip.

There are three stages of hair growth: the anagen phase is the fast growing phase; the involution phase is called the catagen phase; and the third phase is the telogen phase, which is the rest phase.

There are three specific types of hair.

- Lanugo hairs – these are fetal hairs.
- Vellus hairs – infant hairs and fine body hair.
- The final type – the coarse hair type – is called terminal hair.

The distribution of the hair differs between the sexes after puberty has occurred.

The arrector pili muscles are small muscles attached to hair follicles (Figure 51.1). They extend from the dermal coat of the hair follicle to the papillary layer of the dermis. It is this muscle that causes goose bumps (the cholinergic sympathetic supply). The portion where the arrector pili muscle inserts is called the bulge area and it is thought that at this location the stem cells responsible for the regeneration of the hair follicle are located.

The nails

The nails participate in grasping and handling of small things. Nails are highly versatile tools that protect the fingertip, contribute to tactile sensation by acting as a counterforce to the fingertip pad and aid in peripheral thermoregulation via glomus bodies located in the nail bed and matrix (Figure 51.2).

Nails are plates of very tightly packed, hard, keratinised epidermal cells; they develop from the thickened areas of epidermis located at the tips of fingers, thumbs and toes known as nail fields. The nail fields travel on to the dorsal surface surrounded on both sides by folds of epidermis known as nail folds. They are usually located on the dorsal aspect of each distal phalanx. The nail consists of a nail root, the portion of the nail under the skin, a nail body, the visible pink aspect of the nail, the white crescent located at the base of the nail called the lunula, the hyponychium which secures the nail to the finger, the cuticle or eponychium which is a narrow band around the proximal edge of the nail, and a free edge – this is the white end that can extend past the finger.

The almost transparent nail plate combined with the thin epithelium of the nail bed provide a useful way of observing the amount of oxygen present in the blood by revealing the colour of blood in the dermal vessels.

Nails are growing continuously; however, the rate at which they grow slows down as a person ages and if there is evidence of poor circulation. Fingernails grow faster than toenails; the growth rate of a fingernail is said to be in the region of 1–3 mm every 4 weeks while toenails grow about 1 mm per month and take 12–18 months to be completely replaced. Complete nail plate growth may take approximately 6 months. There are some factors that will increase the rate of growth; these include longer digits, summer months, young persons (those less than 30 years) and if the person bites their nails.

The glands

The glands play a key role in the regulation of body temperature. There are three main types of glands associated with the skin:

- sebaceous glands
- sudoriferous glands
- ceruminous glands.

The sebaceous glands

These are oil-secreting glands located in the dermis which secrete sebum. Sebaceous glands are found over most of the surface of the body but are not present on the palms of the hands or the soles of the feet. Sebum helps to prevent hairs from becoming too dry and brittle and the skin from becoming too dry (by preventing excessive evaporation of water from the skin's surface); it also restricts the growth and development of certain bacteria.

The sudoriferous glands

The sudoriferous glands (also known as sweat glands) are divided into two main types. Eccrine glands' ducts terminate at a sweat pore at the outer surface of the epidermis; these are the most common type and their key function is to regulate body temperature by evaporation. Eccrine glands are located throughout the skin except for the margins of the lips, the tympanic membrane and the nail beds of the finger and toenails. Apocrine glands are responsible for 'cold sweats' associated with stressful experiences; their ducts open in hair follicles and they are found in the axillae, the pubic regions and the areola of the breasts.

The ceruminous glands

These glands are located in subcutaneous tissue below the dermis; they secrete cerumen (ear wax) into the ear canal. Cerumen, along with the hairs in the outer ear, protects the ear from particles originating outside the body, for example dust, fine sand or similar. Cerumen provides a sticky barrier preventing many such particles from going further into the ear.

Clinical practice point

Usually hair loss (alopecia) is not something to be concerned about, but occasionally it can be a sign of a medical condition. Some types of hair loss are permanent, for example male and female pattern baldness, which is often hereditary (it runs in the family). Other types of hair loss may be temporary. Hair loss can be caused by an illness, stress, some forms of cancer treatment, weight loss and iron deficiency. Hair loss from cancer treatment can affect people in a number of ways. Some treatments may only cause partial hair loss or thinning, whilst others cause loss of hair from all over the body. Different types of chemotherapeutic drugs have varying effects, while radiotherapy causes hair loss only in the area where treatment is focused. Treating thinning hair carefully can also prevent further hair loss.

Scalp cooling may help to reduce hair loss from the head caused by some chemotherapy drugs. Scalp cooling can reduce the blood flow to the scalp which can stop the chemotherapeutic drug from affecting the hair. It is not always possible to know how well it will work until the person tries it. Scalp cooling is not suitable during treatment for some types of cancer.

52 Epithelialisation

Figure 52.1 Epidermal and deep wound healing.

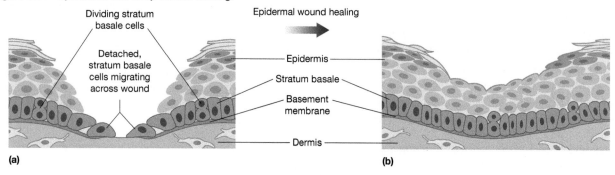

Epidermal wound healing

(a)
- Dividing stratum basale cells
- Detached, stratum basale cells migrating across wound

(b)
- Epidermis
- Stratum basale
- Basement membrane
- Dermis

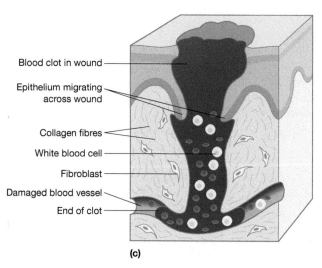

- Blood clot in wound
- Epithelium migrating across wound
- Collagen fibres
- White blood cell
- Fibroblast
- Damaged blood vessel
- End of clot

(c)

Deep wound healing

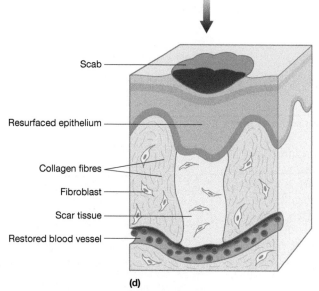

- Scab
- Resurfaced epithelium
- Collagen fibres
- Fibroblast
- Scar tissue
- Restored blood vessel

(d)

Source: Peate I, Wild K & Nair M (eds). Nursing Practice: Knowledge and Care (2014).

Anatomy and Physiology for Nursing and Healthcare Students at a Glance, Second Edition. Ian Peate.
© 2022 John Wiley & Sons Ltd. Published 2022 by John Wiley & Sons Ltd.
Companion website: www.wiley.com/go/peate/anatomyandphysiology

Epithelialisation is the body's physiological response to healing in its attempt to restore and maintain homeostasis. It is characterised by the proliferation and migration of epithelial cells across the wound surface. Epithelialisation usually occurs in response to tissue damage, for example after a wound has occurred.

Wounds

A wound is a breakdown in the protective functions provided by the skin where there is loss of continuity of the epithelium. This may or may not include the underlying connective tissue, for example, the muscle, bone or nerve after an injury to the skin has occurred that may be caused by surgery, direct trauma, a cut, chemicals, heat/cold, friction/shear force, pressure or as a result of pathology (for example, cancer).

Wounds can be described in a number of ways; by the cause (aetiology), anatomical location, whether the wound is acute or chronic, by the method of closure (primary, secondary or delayed closure), by presenting symptoms or by the appearance of the predominant tissue types in the wound bed.

The goal in wound management is to restore structure and function and enhance the cosmetic appearance as quickly as possible. Injuries that occur to the epidermis are epidermal wounds; deeper wounds penetrate and enter the dermis.

How wounds heal

When a wound has occurred (damage to the skin), this sets in motion a range of activities that set out to achieve the goals associated with wound management and to re-establish skin integrity. The wound has only two mechanisms by which it can heal: tissue regeneration or tissue repair.

All wounds heal by two independent methods: contraction and epithelialisation.

Contraction occurs as a wound heals, producing a bed of granulation tissues and causing the edges of the wound to contract. This eventually covers the surface of the wound.

Epithelialisation is a complex process associated with cell proliferation. As cells proliferate, they migrate to cover the surface of the cutaneous defect.

The epidermis has the capacity to regenerate identical cells; in superficial damage when the basal layer of the dermis is still intact, normal anatomical structure and function are restored quickly.

When the injury extends deeper, penetrating the dermis and causing damage to some of the intricate structures, for example the hair follicles, sweat glands, nerve and blood vessels, then more complex biological processes are needed to carry out tissue repair. The anatomical structure and function (depending on the extent of damage) may not be restored. Figure 52.1 shows epidermal and deep wound healing.

Types of wound healing

Primary closure

This is sometimes known as healing by primary intention; healing follows minimal damage to tissues where the borders of the wound are in close opposition. This involves re-epithelialisation as the outer layer closes over the wound. Cells grow in from the margins of the wound and out from epithelial cells, lining the hair follicles and sweat glands.

Inflammation occurs where the surfaces have been cut, while blood clot formation and cell debris fill the breach between the edges. Phagocytes begin to remove the clots and cell debris, encouraging fibroblast activity. Collagen fibres are secreted by the fibroblasts, beginning to bring the surfaces together.

Epithelial cells proliferate across the wound; the epidermis meets and grows upwards, ceasing when full thickness has occurred. The clot formed becomes a scab.

Wounds where the borders are in close opposition (well approximated) are those that can be closely aligned, for example a surgical incision. In the case of a surgical incision, the edges of the wound are mechanically brought together without tension. Closure can occur using butterfly sutures (adhesive strips), sutures, glue (skin adhesives), clips or staples. As there is no loss of tissue, and if there is no risk of infection, the healing process in this case is quick. Often these types of wound heal in 4–21 days and result in minimal scarring and the best aesthetic appearance.

Secondary closure

Wounds that heal by secondary closure, where primary closure is not possible, may involve some degree of tissue loss and the margins of the wound cannot be approximated. A wound's depth can be described as partial thickness or full thickness. As wounds heal by secondary intention, the wound fills with granulation tissue and re-epithelialisation occurs, principally from the wound edges, and eventually a scar forms. These wounds take longer to heal and can often cause scarring.

Delayed primary closure

Delayed primary closure can also be called tertiary wound closure. Wounds in this category are intentionally kept open to allow local conditions such as oedema or infection to abate or to allow the elimination of exudate. As conditions improve, these wounds are later closed using sutures or other procedures.

Wound closure

Wound closure occurs when a number of processes come together. These include granulation, contraction and epithelialisation.

The final stage of wound healing is epithelialisation. This occurs when the germinal layer of the epidermis (stratum basale) responds to chemical signals to proliferate and migrate across the granulation tissue with the intention of forming a new layer of epidermal cells. When this occurs, a new basement membrane and dermoepidermal junction are created and the neoepidermis maintains proliferation and differentiates into the stratified, cornified epithelium (stratum corneum) of normal skin. There is active division, migration and maturation of epidermal cells from the wound edges across the open wound. Speedy epithelialisation is dependent upon a source of epidermal cells, a wound bed that is composed of healthy granulation tissue and a favourable wound microenvironment. Epithelialisation progresses depending upon the size of the wound and how it changes over time.

Clinical practice point

Aseptic non-touch technique (ANTT) refers to the technique and precautions implemented during clinical procedures with the aim of protecting the patient from infection by preventing the transfer of micro-organisms to the patient from the healthcare worker, their equipment or the environment. ANTT must be applied to all clinical procedures which bypass the body's natural defences, for example inserting or accessing intravenous devices, phlebotomy, urinary catheterisation and applying or changing wound dressings. When carrying out ANTT in a person's own home, the healthcare professional must adapt the procedure to ensure the environment is conducive.

The key principles of ANTT are as follows.

A – Always ensure hands are decontaminated effectively prior to the procedure
N – Never contaminate key parts of sterile materials/equipment of the patient's susceptible key sites
T – Touch non-key parts with confidence
T – Take appropriate Infection Prevention and Control precautions at all times

53 Granulation

Figure 53.1 Summary of wound healing events.

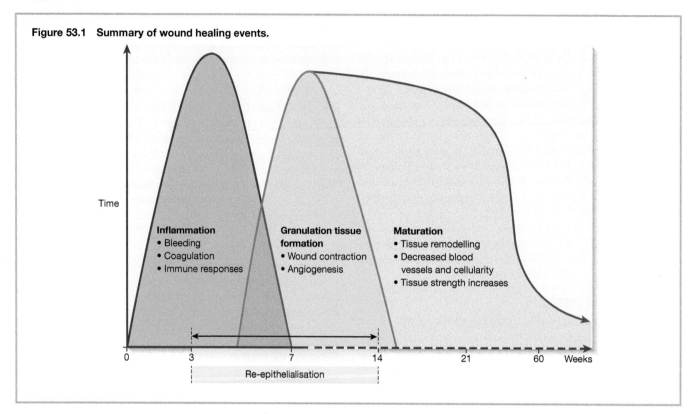

Granulation is an essential physiological requirement that is required for wound healing; other wound healing factors include epithelialisation (see Chapter 52) and contraction. Figure 53.1 provides a summary of wound healing events.

Granulation tissue

Tissue granulation occurs in the proliferative phase of the process of wound healing, during which new, healthy tissue reforms and rebuilds the area of the wound. Granulation tissue is composed of a newly formed wound matrix – containing collagen, matrix proteins and proteoglycans – that forms at the site of an injury. This collagen matrix offers the scaffolding (structural strength) into which new capillaries grow. During granulation, the skin cells are most active; granulation tissue is actively growing connective tissue.

Angiogenesis (the creation of new blood vessels and in this instance capillary formation) supports the growth of new connective tissue along with the nourishment of macrophages and collagen-secreting fibroblasts. The presence of hyaluronic acid within the extracellular matrix stimulates the production of cytokines, such as transforming growth factor (TGF), that act on the macrophages to encourage angiogenesis. Macrophages that migrate to the wound are further stimulated into angiogenesis as they come into contact with the hypoxic wound environment that has been caused by damage to the blood supply when injury occurred.

When a wound begins the granulation process, this indicates that the body is starting to rebuild after the injury. Granulation tissue is a highly fibrous tissue that is typically pink as the body produces numerous small capillaries to provide a rich supply of oxygen and nutrients as well as assisting in the removal of waste. Granulation tissue appears bumpy and uneven. As the process begins, granulation tissue may appear reddened and irritated, as a result of the numerous blood vessels that it contains.

The subsequent granulation tissue present in the wound is red in colour and this is often described as granular or grainy in its appearance. The tissue eventually fills up the injury site and a scar may appear; over time this will fade.

The ability of injured tissue to restore itself is contingent on the amount of damage as well as the regenerative capability of that tissue. In large open wounds, for example, the parenchyma (the cells that make up the functioning part of the skin) and the stroma (the supporting connective tissue) become active in tissue repair.

Tissue repair

The success of tissue repair is based on a number of factors including nutrition and blood supply. The process of healing demands much nutritional support, drawing on the body's nutritional stores. As the majority of structural components of tissue are protein, it is essential that the diet contains a sufficient amount of protein. There are also a number of vitamins that play a central role in the healing of wounds and repair of tissue. When there are deficiencies in vitamins, minerals and trace elements, wound healing will be negatively influenced. Under the direct influence of vitamin C are collagen synthesis, the development of the delicate fibrils usually present in collagen fibres of connective tissues (called fibrillogenesis), and angiogenesis. Vitamin B is directly responsible for the production of protein, formation of antibodies, development of granulation tissue and epithelialisation. Vitamin A has a central role in angiogenesis, macrophage mobility and chemotaxis, and also manages some of the negative effects radiation has on wound healing.

Haemoglobin synthesis involves iron and as such oxygenation trace elements, for example, copper and zinc are required for encouraging collagen formation and epithelialisation.

Blood circulation is essential for the transportation of oxygen, nutrients, antibodies and other cells involved in defending the body to the site of injury where granulation and tissue repair are to take place.

Blood removes bacteria, foreign bodies and debris that would otherwise affect the healing process.

When a significant amount of granulation does occur, it usually leaves a visible and wide scar as a result of the difference between the new and the old tissue.

The final phase of wound healing is the remodelling phase, when the new tissue fully integrates with the old tissue. This phase may take weeks, months or years depending on the severity of the wound; in many cases, complete remodelling does not occur and scars remain visible.

Overgranulation

In some instances, an excess of granulation tissue (also called hypergranulation) may be produced which affects the migrating keratinocytes. The presence of such tissue will prevent epithelial migration occurring across the wound, which will lead to delayed wound healing. Granulation continues even when granulation tissue is level with the surrounding skin.

Hypergranulation tissue is usually seen as a pale or light purple uneven mass that rises above the level of the skin. Excessive and extended stimulation of fibroblasts and angiogenesis causes mounds of granulation tissue that will bleed easily and ooze haemoserous exudate. Overgranulation can interfere with the rate of wound healing.

> ### Clinical practice point
>
> A skin graft is where healthy skin is removed from an unaffected area of the body and used to cover lost or damaged skin. Skin grafts can be used for open fractures (where bone breaks the skin), large wounds or where an area of the skin is surgically removed, for example due to cancer or burns.
>
> There are two main types of skin graft. Partial- or split-thickness skin graft is where a thin layer of skin (tissue paper thin) is shaved from an area that usually heals well, for example the thigh, buttocks or calf. The donor area usually takes 2–3 weeks to heal and is pink for a few months before fading to leave a faint (hardly noticeable) scar. Full-thickness grafting is where the full thickness of skin (the top layer and layers underneath) is removed and the area is directly closed. Sites often used include the neck, behind the ear, the upper arm and groin. Because this type of skin graft is thicker, picking up a new blood supply can be more difficult, so any dressing will be left in place for 5–7 days before being removed. Prior to the procedure, a general or local anaesthetic is given depending on the size and location of the affected area. The skin graft is usually held in place by stitches, staples, clips or skin adhesive. The area is covered with a sterile dressing until it has connected with the surrounding blood supply, which takes around 5–7 days. A dressing is also placed over the area from which the skin has been taken (the donor site) to help protect it from infection. The donor area of partial-thickness skin grafts takes around 2 weeks to heal. In full-thickness grafts, the donor area only takes about 5–10 days to heal as it is normally quite small and is closed with stitches.
>
> At first, the grafted area will appear reddish-purple, but this should fade over time. It can take a year or two for the appearance of the skin to settle down completely. The final colour may be slightly different from the surrounding skin and the area may be slightly indented.

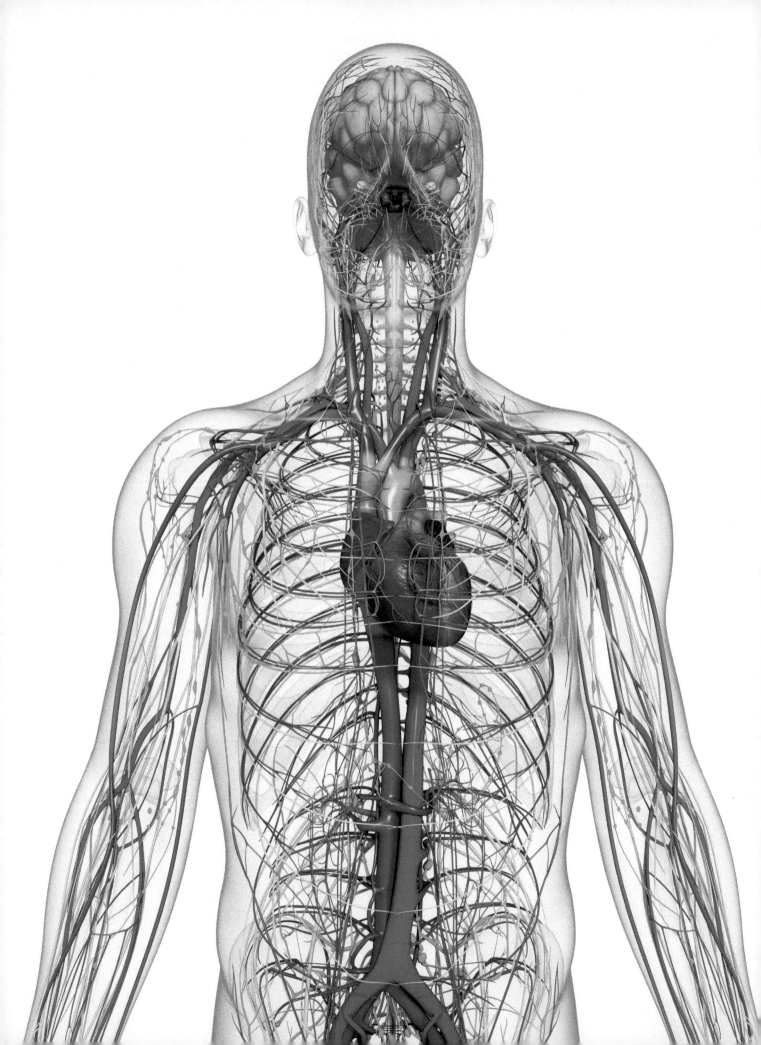

The senses

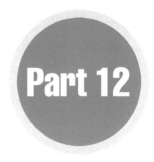

Part 12

Chapters

54 Sight

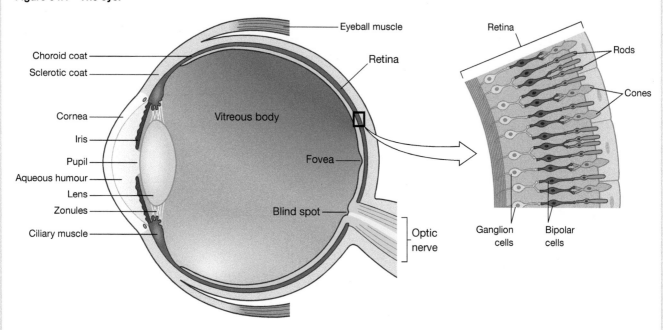

Figure 54.1   The eye.

Eyeball muscle

Choroid coat
Sclerotic coat

Retina

Cornea

Vitreous body

Iris

Pupil

Fovea

Aqueous humour

Lens

Zonules

Blind spot

Ciliary muscle

Optic nerve

Retina

Rods

Cones

Ganglion cells

Bipolar cells

Table 54.1 Structures of the eye.

Structures that protect the eye	Anterior aspect of the eye	Posterior aspect of the eye	The visual system pathways to the brain
• Orbit	• Cornea	• Retina	• Optic nerves and optic tracts
• Eye lids	• Aqueous humour	• Vitreous humour	• Visual cortex
• Eye lashes and eyebrows	• Iris		
• Lacrimal apparatus	• Lens and ciliary muscle		
• Sclera			

Figure 54.2   The lacrimal apparatus.

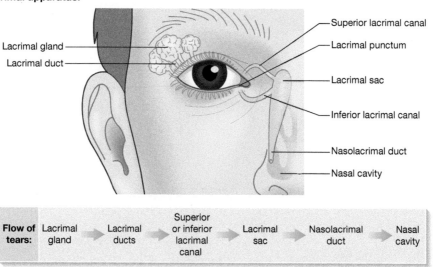

Lacrimal gland

Lacrimal duct

Superior lacrimal canal

Lacrimal punctum

Lacrimal sac

Inferior lacrimal canal

Nasolacrimal duct

Nasal cavity

Flow of tears:	Lacrimal gland	→	Lacrimal ducts	→	Superior or inferior lacrimal canal	→	Lacrimal sac	→	Nasolacrimal duct	→	Nasal cavity

Source: Peate I, Wild K & Nair M (eds). Nursing Practice: Knowledge and Care (2014).

Anatomy and Physiology for Nursing and Healthcare Students at a Glance, Second Edition. Ian Peate.
© 2022 John Wiley & Sons Ltd. Published 2022 by John Wiley & Sons Ltd.
Companion website: www.wiley.com/go/peate/anatomyandphysiology

The special senses are smell, taste, vision and hearing (including equilibrium). They are known as the special senses because their sensory receptors are located within relatively large sensory organs located in the head – the nose, tongue, eyes and ears. The skin is sometimes considered a sense organ (see Part 11: The Skin).

Vision

The eye permits us to see and understand shapes, colours and dimensions of objects by processing the light they reflect or emit. The detects bright or dim light and is scomplex structure. See Table 54.1 for the structures related to the eye.

The eye consists of the cornea, iris, pupil, lens and retina (this houses the light-sensitive photoreceptors) (Figure 54.1).

The orbit

The orbit protects the eye, located at the front of the skull, with a wider opening anteriorly narrowing to a small opening posteriorly where the optic nerve exits, connecting the visual pathways and brain.

Eyelids, lashes, eyebrows

External to the eye ball, these structures provide protection. Other protective structures include the conjunctiva, lacrimal apparatus and extrinsic eye muscles.

Eyelids are thin, loose folds of skin covering the anterior eye, protecting it from foreign bodies and excessive light; they also spread tears by blinking. They contain the puncta through which tears flow. Eyebrows provide shade, keeping perspiration and other debris away from the eyes. Eyelashes protect from foreign particles and act as sensors – an unexpected touch initiates the blinking reflex.

The lacrimal apparatus

The lacrimal apparatus (Figure 54.2) produces and drains lacrimal fluid. The surface of the eye is continuously bathed in tears. The structure secretes, distributes and drains, cleans and moisturises the eye's surface.

Fluid is pumped throughout the system each time blinking occurs. Tears, which have antimicrobial properties, are drained away via the nasolacrimal system.

The sclera

The sclera is derived from interwoven collagen fibrils of varying widths within ground substance maintained by fibroblasts. It is made up from three layers of varying thickness.

The cornea

Transparent to light, the cornea does not contain blood vessels and is approximately 11 mm in diameter and 500 µm thick in the centre. The cornea is more curved than the rest of the globe. With the lens, it transmits and focuses light into the eye and protects the inner ocular structures.

The aqueous humour

This is a transparent fluid that fills the anterior chamber of the eye, providing oxygen and nutrients to the lens and cornea. The aqueous is part of the optical pathway of the eye.

The iris

The iris, the coloured aspect of the eyeball, shaped like a flattened doughnut, controls light levels inside the eye similar to the aperture on a camera. The round opening in the centre is the pupil. A number of tiny muscles embedded in the iris dilate and constrict pupil size.

The circular sphincter muscle lies around the very edge of the pupil, causing it to constrict in bright light. The radial dilator muscle runs radially through the iris, dilating the eye in dim light.

The lens and ciliary muscle

The lens is posterior to the pupil and the iris; it is a transparent structure, changing its shape in order to increase or decrease the amount of refracting power applied to light entering the eye. The lens provides the remaining variable focusing power and serves to further refine the focus, permitting the eye to focus on objects at different distances.

An elastic extracellular matrix, the capsule surrounds the lens providing a smooth optical surface and acting as an anchor for suspension of the lens within the eye. A meshwork of non-elastic microfibrils, or 'zonules', anchors into the capsule close to the equator of the lens, connecting into ciliary muscle. The ciliary muscle is part of the ciliary body, divided into ciliary muscle, ciliary processes and pars plana.

The retina

Mostly this is a transparent thin tissue designed to capture photons of light and initiate processing of the image by the brain. The average thickness of the retina is 250 µm and it consists of 10 layers.

There are two types of receptors in the eye: rods and cones. The outer segment contains light-sensitive visual pigment molecules – opsins – in stacked discs (rods) or invaginations (cones). Cones provide the ability to discern colour and the ability to see fine detail; they are more concentrated in the central retina. Rods are mainly responsible for peripheral vision and vision under low light conditions and are more prevalent in the mid-peripheral and peripheral retina.

Visual system pathways to the brain

The optic nerves meet at the optic chiasma, where axons from the medial half of each retina cross to the opposite side, forming pairs of axons from each eye – the left and right optic tracts. The crossing of the axons results in each optic tract carrying information from both eyes; the left carries visual information from the lateral half of the retina of the left eye and the medial half of the retina of the right eye, whereas the right tract carries visual information from the lateral half of the retina of the right eye and the medial half of the retina of the left eye.

The visual cortex

This is located in the occipital lobe of the brain, where the final processing of neural signals from the retina takes place and vision occurs. The occipital lobe is at the most posterior portion of the brain.

Clinical practice point

Cataracts occur when the lens of the eye develops cloudy patches. As we age, they start to become frosted and begin to limit vision. Usually cataracts will slowly get worse over time. Surgery to replace the cloudy lens is the only way to improve eyesight. There are no medications or eye drops that have been shown to improve cataracts or stop them getting worse.

55 Hearing

Figure 55.1   The ear.

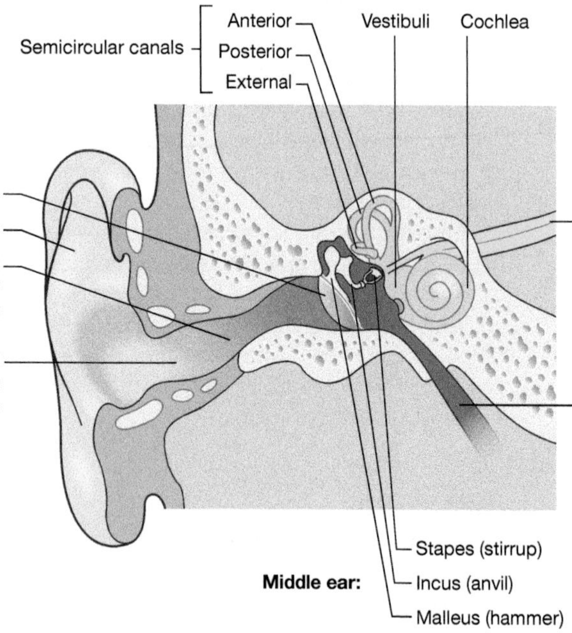

Internal ear:
Anterior
Posterior — Vestibuli   Cochlea
External

Semicircular canals

External ear:
Eardrum
Auricle
External
auditory
meatus

External
acoustic
meatus

Auditory
nerve

Eustachian
tube

Stapes (stirrup)
Middle ear: Incus (anvil)
Malleus (hammer)

Source: Peate I, Wild K & Nair M (eds). Nursing Practice: Knowledge and Care (2014).

Figure 55.2   The outer ear.

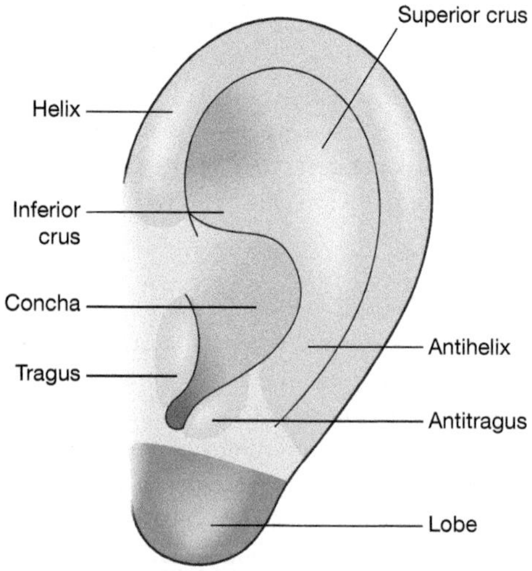

Superior crus

Helix

Inferior
crus

Concha

Tragus

Antihelix

Antitragus

Lobe

Source: Peate I, Wild K & Nair M (eds). Nursing Practice:
Knowledge and Care (2014).

Figure 55.3   The middle ear.

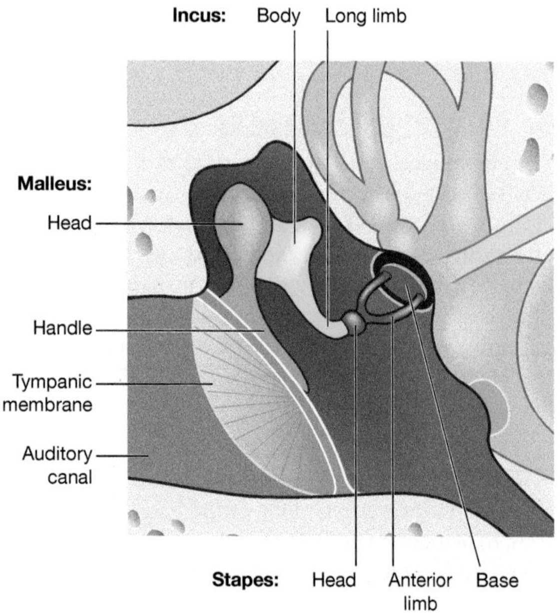

Incus: Body   Long limb

Malleus:
Head

Handle

Tympanic
membrane

Auditory
canal

Stapes: Head   Anterior   Base
limb

Source: Peate I, Wild K & Nair M (eds). Nursing Practice: Knowledge and Care (2014).

Figure 55.4   The inner ear.

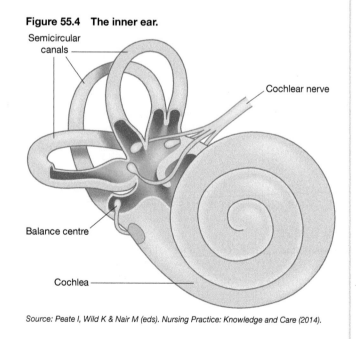

Semicircular
canals

Cochlear nerve

Balance centre

Cochlea

Source: Peate I, Wild K & Nair M (eds). Nursing Practice: Knowledge and Care (2014).

Sound represents a combination of waves generated by a vibrating sound source(s) transmitted through the air until they reach the ear. Wave frequency corresponds to what is perceived as pitch, amplitude corresponds to the loudness or intensity of sound.

The ear

The ear has two key functions: to assist with balance (equilibrium) and to allow us to hear the sounds around us. The ear is composed of three sections (Figure 55.1): outer (external), middle and inner ear.

The outer (external) ear

This aspect of the ear assists with the functions of the middle ear although it is not an anatomical part of it. The auricle and external acoustic meatus (external auditory canal) make up the external ear. The external ear collects and amplifies sound, which is transmitted to the middle ear. The asymmetrical shape introduces delays in the path of sound which assist in sound localisation (Figure 55.2).

The arterial supply is composed of the posterior auricular artery, anterior auricular branch of the superficial temporal artery and occipital artery. Veins accompany corresponding named arteries.

The external ear is supplied by the auriculotemporal (fifth cranial) nerve and contributions from cranial nerves VII, IX and X and the great auricular nerve.

The middle ear

The key function of the middle ear (tympanic cavity) is bony conduction of sound via transference of sound waves in the air collected by the auricle to the fluid of the inner ear. The middle ear sits in the petrous portion of the temporal bone and is filled with air secondary to communication with the nasopharynx via the auditory (eustachian) tube (Figure 55.3).

The middle ear extends from the tympanic membrane to the oval window containing the bony conduction elements of the ossicles. The walls of the tympanic cavity are complex with important associations.

Tympanic membrane

The tympanic membrane is a thin oval, semi-transparent membrane separating the external and middle ears. Air vibrations collected by the auricle are transferred to the mobile tympanic membrane, which then transmits the sound to the ossicles. Multiple structures are contained within the tympanic cavity. Muscles, nerves and the auditory tube occupy space within the tympanic cavity.

Ossicles

From the deep surface of the tympanic membrane to the oval window is a chain of moveable bones, the ossicles – malleus (hammer), incus (anvil) and stapes (stirrup). These transmit and amplify sound waves from the air to the perilymph of the internal ear.

Auditory tube

The auditory tube (eustachian tube) communicates between the middle ear and the nasopharynx. It equalises pressure across the tympanic membrane.

The blood supply is derived from a number of arteries, primarily from the external and internal carotid. The middle ear is supplied by the auriculotemporal (Vth cranial) and tympanic (IXth cranial) nerves and by the auricular branch of the vagus.

The inner ear

The inner ear consists of a membranous labyrinth encased in an osseous labyrinth. The vestibule and semicircular canals are associated with vestibular function (balance). The cochlea, a coiled tube, is concerned with hearing, (Figure 55.4).

A layer of dense bone creates the surface outline of the inner ear. The walls of the bony labyrinth are continuous with the surrounding temporal bone. The inner aspects of the bony labyrinth closely follow the contours of the membranous labyrinth; a delicate, interconnected network of fluid-filled tubes where the receptors are found.

The walls of the bony labyrinth are made up of dense bone, apart from two small areas located close to the cochlear spiral. The round window consists of a thin, membranous partition separating the perilymph of the cochlear chambers from the air-filled middle ear. Collagen fibres connect the bony margins of the oval window at the base of the stapes.

Perilymph, which closely resembles cerebrospinal fluid, flows between the bony and membranous labyrinths. Endolymph is contained in the membranous labyrinth. These fluids are in separate compartments.

The bony labyrinth can be subdivided into the vestibule, three semicircular canals and the cochlea.

The vestibule

This contains a pair of membranous sacs: the saccule and the utricle. Receptors here provide for sensations of gravity and linear acceleration.

The semicircular canals

These enclose the slender semicircular ducts. Receptors are stimulated when the head moves. The fluid-filled chambers within the vestibule are usually continuous with the semicircular canals.

The cochlea

This bony, spiral-shaped chamber contains the cochlear duct of the membranous labyrinth. The sense of hearing is provided by receptors within the cochlear duct. Two perilymph-filled chambers are on either side of the duct.

Blood supply to the inner ear

The internal auditory artery supplies the entire membranous labyrinth, passing through the internal auditory meatus and dividing into three branches. The cochlear artery supplies the entire cochlea via the spiral arteries.

The organ of Corti

This is located in the cochlea and is referred to as the receptor organ of hearing. Hair cells within the organ of Corti sense mechanical forces (inner and outer hair cells); 95% of the afferent fibres are from the inner hair cells, which are the sensory receptors communicating with neurons from the VIIIth cranial nerve. Outer hair cells receive efferent input.

Clinical practice point

Ménière's disease is a condition of the inner ear. A person with Ménière's disease may experience vertigo, become unsteady on their feet, feel nauseous or vomit, hear ringing, roaring or buzzing inside the ear (tinnitus) or have a sudden drop in hearing. These symptoms often happen all at once and can last minutes or hours (2–3 hours). The condition usually starts in one ear but can spread to both ears over time. It may take a day or two for the symptoms to disappear completely. After the attack, the person may feel tired. Symptoms will vary from person to person but an episode of hearing loss without vertigo is uncommon. The events can occur in clusters, several times a week, or they may be separated by weeks, months or years. Ménière's disease most commonly affects those aged 20–60 years. There is no cure but medication can help control the vertigo, nausea and vomiting. The aim is to provide medication for the symptoms as soon as possible. Treatment may be required for tinnitus, hearing loss and loss of balance.

56 Olfaction

Figure 56.1 Pathway of smell.

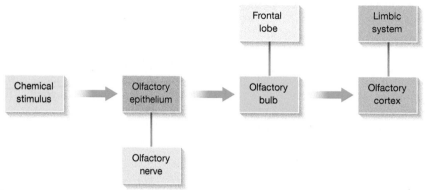

Figure 56.2 Olfactory epithelium and olfactory receptor cells.

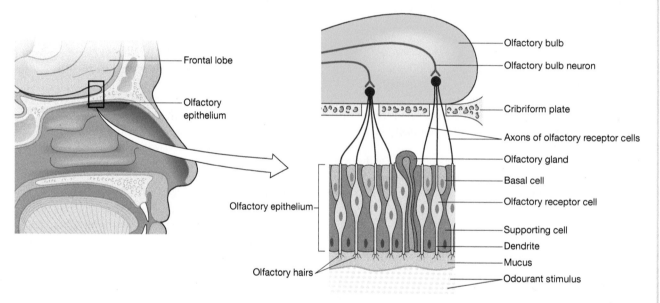

Figure 56.3 The olfactory bulb (nerve).

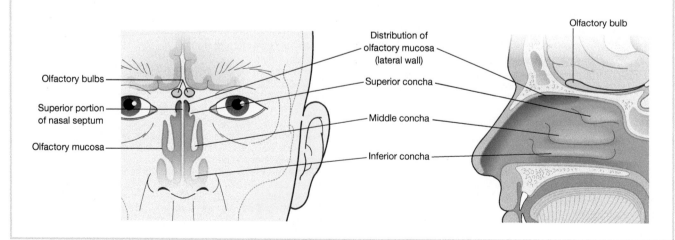

Anatomy and Physiology for Nursing and Healthcare Students at a Glance, Second Edition. Ian Peate.
© 2022 John Wiley & Sons Ltd. Published 2022 by John Wiley & Sons Ltd.
Companion website: www.wiley.com/go/peate/anatomyandphysiology

Olfaction refers to the sense of smell (along with taste) which is a chemical sense. The sensations come from the interaction of molecules with smell receptors. Some smells can evoke strong emotional responses as the impulse for smell spreads to the limbic system (Figure 56.1). When a person is constantly exposed to an odour, the perception of the odour will diminish and cease within minutes; the loss of perception only involves that specific odour.

With the sense of smell we are able to evaluate our environment, taking in a large amount of information. We are always assessing the air that we inhale, which can alert us to possible dangers, for example, the presence of smoke. Smell also enables us to decipher other important information, such as the quality of food – if it is edible or potentially poisonous (rotten or gone off) – as well as being able to identify the presence of another being; it also influences social and sexual behaviour. Humans have an innate ability to detect bad, unpleasant, dangerous smells. The sense of smell is important for survival and quality of life.

Physiology of olfaction

The nose contains between 10 and 100 million olfactory receptor neurons. These occur in the olfactory epithelium lining the mucosa in the nasal cavity.

The olfactory system starts with olfactory receptor cells situated in the nasal epithelium of the nasal cavity (Figure 56.2). Above this is a layer of protective bone. Axons of the olfactory receptor cells merge to form the olfactory nerves. The ends of the axons form spherical glomeruli, each of which receives input from the same olfactory receptor. The glomerular layer is permeated by dendrites from mitral cell neurons, which in turn transmit information to the olfactory bulb, located in the cerebral cortex.

Specialised receptor cells (olfactory receptor neurons) of the olfactory epithelium in the nose detect smells. Olfaction relies on the binding of odourant molecules to receptors located on the receptor cells. Olfaction has complex systems of coding, displaying differing methods for coding the receptor stimulus. There are numerous central projections that allow for the perception and interpretation of important sensory inputs.

Located in the roof of each nostril is the nasal mucosa. This contains the olfactory epithelium, which is covered by mucus. As well as the sensory cells, the epithelium contains Bowman's glands which produce the secretion that saturates the surface of the receptors. This aqueous secretion contains mucopolysaccharides, immunoglobulins, proteins (such lysozyme) and various enzymes.

A pigmented type of epithelial cell is also located in the nasal mucosa (membrane); the reason for its pigmentation is unknown. The nasal epithelium contains the receptor cells, possessing a terminal enlargement above the epithelial surface, with approximately 8–20 olfactory cilia which contain the smell receptors.

Olfactory nerve and cribriform plate

Small, unmyelinated axons of the olfactory receptor cells form the fine fibres of the first cranial nerve and travel centrally toward the ipsilateral olfactory bulb, making contact with the second-order neurons. The trigeminal nerve (cranial nerve V) sends fibres to the olfactory epithelium detecting caustic chemicals, such as ammonia. The cribriform plate of the ethmoid bone, separated at the midline by the crista galli, comprises a number of small foramina; the olfactory nerve fibres traverse this.

Olfactory bulb

The olfactory bulb lies below the basal frontal lobe and is a highly organised structure composed of several distinct layers and synaptic specialisations (Figure 56.3). The layers are:

- glomerular layer
- external plexiform layer
- mitral cell layer
- internal plexiform layer
- granule cell layer.

Olfactory tract

Mitral cell axons project into the olfactory cortex via the olfactory tract. Medial fibres of the tract contact the anterior olfactory nucleus and the septal area. There are some fibres that project to the contralateral olfactory bulb via the anterior commissure.

It is assumed that the thalamic connections serve as a conscious mechanism for odour perception, while the amygdala and the entorhinal area are limbic system components and might be involved in the affective mechanisms of olfaction.

Clinical practice point

Rhinoplasty (nose reshaping) is a surgical procedure undertaken to change the shape or size of the nose for cosmetic reasons or to help the person breathe more easily. Rhinoplasty is usually carried out under general anaesthetic Depending on the type of surgery, the nose may be made smaller (nose reduction), by removing some of the cartilage and bone, or to make the nose larger (nose augmentation), by taking cartilage from the ears and bone from the hips, elbow or skull and using this to build up the nose. The shape of the nose (including the nostrils) can be changed by breaking the nose bone and rearranging the cartilage. It is also possible to change the angle between the nose and top lip. The skin over the nose should shrink or expand to its new shape. The procedure involves either making a cut across the skin between the nostrils (open rhinoplasty) or small cuts inside the nostrils (closed rhinoplasty). A closed rhinoplasty will leave no visible scars and causes less swelling. The procedure can take 1.5–3 hours and it is usual for the person to stay in hospital for 1–2 nights. A dressing is applied to the nose for the first 12 hours postoperatively and a splint held over the nose with tape for 7 days. The person may not be able to breathe through their nose for about a week. Analgesia is given to help control any pain or discomfort.

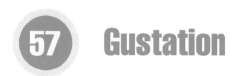

57 Gustation

Figure 57.1   The tongue.

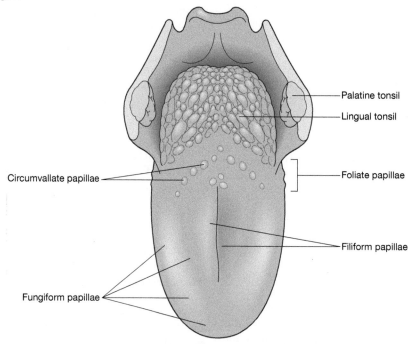

Palatine tonsil

Lingual tonsil

Circumvallate papillae

Foliate papillae

Filiform papillae

Fungiform papillae

Figure 57.2   Taste.

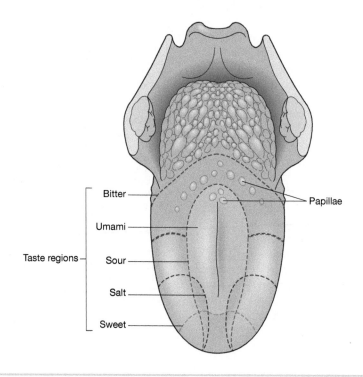

Bitter

Umami

Papillae

Taste regions

Sour

Salt

Sweet

Anatomy and Physiology for Nursing and Healthcare Students at a Glance, Second Edition. Ian Peate.
© 2022 John Wiley & Sons Ltd. Published 2022 by John Wiley & Sons Ltd.
Companion website: www.wiley.com/go/peate/anatomyandphysiology

The word 'gustation' comes from the Latin *gustationem*, meaning taste or like; it is the formal term for the sense of taste. In order to create the sensation of taste, a substance has to be in a solution of saliva so that the substance can enter the taste pores.

Taste drives the appetite and can also help to protect the person from poison. Mostly when a person tastes bitter or sour, this causes dislike because most poisons are bitter, whilst foods that have gone off can taste acidic.

The tongue

The tongue is a muscular organ in the mouth and is covered with moist, pink tissue called mucosa; it is a boneless mass that the person can, at will, fold, invert, lay flat or poke out of the mouth. It is the papillae that give the tongue its rough texture. Thousands of taste buds cover the surfaces of the papillae (Figure 57.1).

Anatomy and physiology

The taste bud, located on the tongue, is the functional unit that permits us to discriminate between the tastes of sweet, sour, salty and bitter. There are over 100 taste receptor cells in each taste bud.

The sense of taste is mediated by groups of taste buds, which sample oral concentrations of a large number of small molecules and report a sensation of taste to centres located in the brainstem. The papillae are projections of a connective tissue core that is covered with squamous epithelium. The types of papilla are circumvallate (vallate), foliate, fungiform and filiform (Figure 57.2).

The taste buds are so small that they cannot be seen by the naked eye and a microscope is required to visualise them. However, the papillae can be observed by close inspection of the surface of the tongue. The fungiform papillae stand out clearly. The taste buds have a life span of approximately 10–12 days.

As well as signal transduction by taste buds, the sense of smell is also profoundly affected by the sensation of taste.

The sense of taste is caused by the excitation of taste receptors and receptors for a large number of particular chemicals have been recognised that influence the reception of taste. These include receptors for such chemicals as sodium, potassium, chloride, glutamate and adenosine. Five categories of tastes are generally recognised:

* salty
* sour
* sweet
* bitter
* umami.

Monosodium glutamate is the taste of umami which has recently been recognised as a unique taste as it cannot be elicited by any amalgamation of the four other taste types. Glutamate is present in a number of protein-rich foods and is particularly abundant in ripened cheese.

The perception of taste appears to be influenced by thermal stimulation of the tongue. For some people, warming the front of the tongue creates a clear sweet sensation and cooling leads to a salty or sour sensation. None of the tastes are elicited by a single chemical.

Taste bud anatomy

Taste buds are made up of groups of around 40 columnar epithelial cells that are bundled together along their long axes. The taste cells within a bud are arranged in such a way that their tips form a small taste pore and through this pore extend microvilli from the taste cells. The microvilli of the taste cells contain taste receptors and it has been suggested that most taste buds contain cells that have receptors for two or three of the basic tastes.

Intertwined among the taste cells in a taste bud is a system of dendrites of sensory nerves that are called taste nerves. When the binding of chemicals to their receptors stimulates taste cells, they depolarise and this depolarisation is spread to the taste nerve fibres, resulting in an action potential that is eventually transmitted to the brain. This nerve transmission rapidly adapts; after the first stimulus, a powerful discharge is seen in the taste nerve fibres but within a few seconds the response reduces to a steady-state level at a much lower amplitude.

When the taste signals are transmitted to the brain, a number of efferent neural pathways are activated, which are important to digestive function. Tasting food, for example, is followed very quickly by increased salivation and also by low-level secretory activity in the stomach.

Taste preferences often change in conjunction with the needs of the body. For example, we like the taste of sugar as we have an absolute need for carbohydrates; we get cravings for salt because we have to have sodium chloride present in the diet.

Clinical Practice Point

The decreased ability to taste certain types of foods is known as hypogeusia; the absence of taste entirely is termed ageusia. Dysgeusia refers to the presence of a metallic, rancid or foul taste in the mouth. Taking certain medications can also interfere with the ability to taste. While the precise cause of smell dysfunction is not entirely understood, the mostly likely cause is damage to the cells that support and assist the olfactory neurons, called sustentacular cells. Loss of the ability to smell something is called anosmia. The sensations of taste and smell are related, so many disorders of the sense of taste are associated with a decreased or impaired sense of smell. These taste disorders can range from obstructions in or damage to the nose to damage to the brain and nervous system. The most common pure taste disorder is a phantom taste sensation; this is the perception of a bad taste in the mouth that will not go away. Some loss of taste sensation also occurs as part of the normal ageing process and some elderly people may complain of decreased ability to taste foods. Sometimes, having a cold, sinusitis, throat infection or upper respiratory tract infection can result in a decrease in taste sensation. A loss or change to the sense of smell or taste could be caused by COVID-19. A large proportion of people who have tested positive for COVID-19 have reported problems with their sense of smell and taste.

Appendix 1: Normal physiological values

This is a selection of reference ranges for haematological and biochemical investigations. The local laboratory must always be consulted, as ranges differ between laboratories. This list is given for educational purposes only and must not be used for clinical decision making.

Full blood count

Haemoglobin (Hb):

- 130–180 g/L male
- 115–165 g/L female

White cell count (WCC):

- Total: $3.6–11.0 \times 10^9$/L
- Neutrophils: $1.8–7.5 \times 10^9$/L
- Lymphocytes: $1.0–4.0 \times 10^9$/L
- Monocytes: $0.2–0.8 \times 10^9$/L
- Eosinophils: $0.1–0.4 \times 10^9$/L
- Basophils: $0.02–0.10 \times 10^9$/L

Platelet count: $140–400 \times 10^9$/L
Red cell count (RCC):

- $4.5–6.5 \times 10^9$/L male
- $3.8–5.8 \times 10^9$/L female

Haematocrit:

- 0.40–0.54 L/L male
- 0.37–0.47 L/L female

Mean cell volume (MCV): 80–100 fL
Mean corpuscular haemoglobin (MCH): 27–32 pg/cell
Reticulocyte count: 0.2–2%

Coagulation

Prothrombin time (PT): 10–14 seconds
Activated partial thromboplastin time (APTT): 24–37 seconds
Fibrinogen: 1.50–4.50 g/L
D-dimer: less than 500 ng/mL

Haematinics

Ferritin:

- 25–350 ng/mL male
- 10–300 ng/mL female

Vitamin B12: 180–1000 pg/mL
Folate: greater than 4.0 ng/mL
Total serum iron:

- 11.6–35.0 µmol/L male
- 4.6–30.4 µmol/L female

Transferrin: 2.0–3.6 g/L
Transferrin saturation: 20–50%
Total iron binding capacity (TIBC): 45–81 µmol/L

Erythrocyte sedimentation rate (ESR):

- Less than or equal to 49 years: 1–7 male, 3–9 female
- Less than or equal to 50 years: 2–10 male, 5–15 female

Biochemistry

Urea and electrolytes (U&Es)

- Na+: 133–146 mmol/L
- K+: 3.5–5.3 mmol/L
- Ca^{2+}(adjusted): 2.2-2.6 mmol/L
- Mg^{2+}: 0.7–1.0 mmol/L
- Chloride: 98-106 mmol/L
- Urea: 2.5–7.8 mmol/L

Creatinine:

- 59–104 µmol/L male
- 45–84 µmol/ L female

Liver function tests (LFTs)
Alkaline phosphatase (ALP): 30–130 U/L
Alanine aminotransferase (ALT):

- Less than 41 U/L male
- Less than 33 U/L female

Bilirubin: less than 21 µmol/L
Gamma glutamyl transferase (GGT:

- Less than 60 U/L male
- Less than 40 U/L female

Albumin: 35–50 g/L
Inflammatory markers
C-reactive protein (CRP): less than 5 mg/L
Arterial blood gas results
pH: 7.35–7.45
pO_2: 11–13 kPa (82.5–97.5 mmHg)
pCO_2: 4.7–6.0 kPa (35.2–45 mmHg)
HCO_3: 22–26 mmol/L
Base excess: -2 to +2 mmol/L
Metabolic tests
Serum ketones: less than 0.6 mmol/L
Fasting blood glucose: 4.0–6.0 mmol/L
Postprandial (2 hours after eating): up to 7.8 mmol/L
HbA1c: less than 42 mmol/mol (6.0%)
Cholesterol: less than 5 mmol/L
Triglyceride: 0.55–1.90 mmol/L
Low-denisty lipoprotein (LDL): less than 3 mmol/L
High-density lipoprotein (HDL): greater than 1 mmol/L
Cholesterol/HDL: less than 4

Endocrinology

Thyroid-stimulating hormone (TSH): 0.4–4.0 mU/L[2]
Free T4: 9–24 pmol/L
Free T3: 3.5–7.8 pmol/L

Anatomy and Physiology for Nursing and Healthcare Students at a Glance, Second Edition. Ian Peate.
© 2022 John Wiley & Sons Ltd. Published 2022 by John Wiley & Sons Ltd.
Companion website: www.wiley.com/go/peate/anatomyandphysiology

Parathyroid hormone: 10–65 ng/L
Growth hormone (random):

- Less than 5 ng/mL male
- Less than 10 ng/mL female

Cortisol (random): 137–429 nmol/L

Testosterone:

- Male less than 50: 10-45 nmol/L
- Male more than 50: 6.2–26 nmol/L

Triglyceride: 0.55–1.90 mmol/L
LDL: less than 3 mmol/L
HDL: greater than 1 mmol/L
Cholesterol/HDL: less than 4

Other biochemistry tests

Serum total protein: 60–78 g/L
Troponin T: less than 0.01 µg/L
Creatine kinase (CK):

- 40–320 U/L male
- 25–200 U/L female

Lactate dehydrogenase (LDH): 240–480 U/L
Lactate (plasma): 0.5–2.2 mmol/L
Urate:

- 200–430 µmol/L male
- 140–360 µmol/L female

Amylase: 28–100 U/dL
Ammonia: 10–35 µmol/L

B-type natriuretic peptide (NT-proBNP):

- Less than 75 years: less than 125 pg/mL
- Greater than 75 years: less than 450 pg/mL

Copper: 70–150 µg/dL
Ceruloplasmin: 15–60 µmol/L
Vitamin D: greater than 500 nmol/L
Serum osmolality: 275–295 mOsmol/kg
24h urine osmolality: 500–800 mOsm/kg
Random urine osmolality: 300–900 mOsm/kg
12h fluid restricted urine osmolality: greater than 850 mOsm/kg
24h urine sodium (Na+): 100–260 mmol/24h
24h urine potassium (K+): 25–100 mmol/24h
24h urine total protein: less than 100 mg/24h
Urine pH (random): 5–7

Tumour markers

Beta human chorionic gonadotrophin (bHCG): less than 5 m U/mL
Alpha-fetoprotein: less than 44 ng/mL
Prostate specific antigen (PSA): less than 4.0 ng/mL

Carcinoembryonic antigen (CEA):

- Non-smokers at 50 years: less than 3.6 µg/L
- Non-smokers at 70 years: less than 4.1 µg/L
- Smokers: less than 5 µg/L

CA-125: less than 35 U/mL
CA19-9: less than 40 U/mL

Immunology

Anti-SS-A (La):

- Negative: less than 3 U/mL
- Positive: greater than 4 U/mL

Anti-streptolysin O titre (ASOT):

- Pre-school age: less than 100
- School age: less than 250
- Adults: less than 125

Rheumatoid factor (RF):

- Negative: less than 20 U/mL
- Positive: greater than 30 U/mL

Antimitochondrial antibodies (AMA):

- Negative: less than 10 U/mL
- Positive: greater than 10 U/mL

Perinuclear antineutrophil cytoplasmic antibodies (p-ANCA):

- Negative: less than 5 U/mL
- Positive: greater than 5 U/mL

Anti-histone antibodies:

- Negative: less than 25 U/mL
- Positive: greater than 25 U/mL

IgA: 110–560 mg/dL
IgD: 0.5–3.0 mg/dL
IgE: 0.01–0.04 mg/dL
IgG: 800–1800 mg/dL
IgM: 54–200 mg/dL
Anti-ds-DNA:

- Negative: less than 40 U/mL
- Positive: greater than 60 U/mL

Anti-ss-DNA:

- Negative: less than 8 U/mL
- Positive: greater than 10 U/mL

Cytoplasmic antineutrophil cytoplasmic antibodies (c-ANCA):

- Negative: less than 20 U/mL
- Positive: greater than 30 U/mL

Anti-SS-A (Ro):

- Negative: less than 15 U/mL
- Positive: greater than 25 U/mL

Lumbar puncture results

Appearance: clear and colourless
White blood cells (WBC): 0–5 cells/µL

- No neutrophils present, primarily lymphocytes
- Normal cell counts do not rule out meningitis or any other pathology

Red blood cells (RBC): 0–10/mm³
Protein: 0.15–0.45 g/L (or less than 1% of the serum protein concentration)
Glucose: 2.8–4.2 mmol/L (or same or more than 60% plasma glucose concentration)
Opening pressure: 10–20 cmH$_2$O

Appendix 2: Prefixes and suffixes

Prefix: A prefix is positioned at the beginning of a word to modify or change its meaning. Pre means "before." Prefixes may also indicate a location, number, or time.

Suffix: The ending part of a word that changes the meaning of the word.

Prefix or suffix	Meaning	Example(s)
a-, an-	not, without	Analgesic, apathy
ab-	from; away from	Abduction
abdomin(o)-	Of or relating to the abdomen	Abdomen
acous(io)-	Of or relating to hearing	Acoumeter, acoustician
acr(o)-	extremity, topmost	Acrocrany, acromegaly, acroosteolysis, acroposthia
ad-	at, increase, on, toward	Adduction
aden(o)-, aden(i)-	Of or relating to a gland	Adenocarcinoma, adenology, adenotome, adenotyphus
adip(o)-	Of or relating to fat or fatty tissue	Adipocyte
adren(o)-	Of or relating to adrenal glands	Adrenal artery
-aemia	blood condition	Anaemia
aer(o)-	air, gas	Aerosinusitis
aesthesio-	sensation	Aesthesia
anaes-	sensation	Anaesthesia
alb-	Denoting a white or pale colour	Albino
alge(si)-	pain	Analgesic
-algia, alg(i)o-	pain	Myalgia
all(o-)	Denoting something as different, or as an addition	Alloantigen, allopathy
ambi-	Denoting something as positioned on both sides; describing both of two	Ambidextrous
amni-	Pertaining to the membranous fetal sac (amnion)	Amniocentesis
an-	not, without	Analgesia
ana-	back, again, up	Anaplasia
andr(o)-	pertaining to a man	Android, andrology
angi(o)-	blood vessel	Angiogram
ankyl(o)-, ancyl(o)-	Denoting something as crooked or bent	Ankylosis
ante-	Describing something as positioned in front of another thing	Antepartum
anti-	Describing something as 'against' or 'opposed to' another	Antibody, antipsychotic
arteri(o)-	Of or pertaining to an artery	Arteriole, artery
arthr(o)-	Of or pertaining to the joints, limbs	Arthritis
articul(o)-	joint	Articulation
-ase	enzyme	Lactase
-asthenia	weakness	Myasthenia gravis
ather(o)-	fatty deposit, soft gruel-like deposit	Atherosclerosis
atri(o)-	an atrium (esp. heart atrium)	Atrioventricular
aur(i)-	Of or pertaining to the ear	Aural
aut(o)-	self	Autoimmune
axill-	Of or pertaining to the armpit (uncommon as a prefix)	Axilla
bi-	twice, double	Binary
bio-	life	Biology
blephar(o)-	Of or pertaining to the eyelid	Blepharoplast
brachi(o)-	Of or relating to the arm	Brachium of inferior colliculus
brady-	'slow'	Bradycardia
bronch(i)-	bronchus	Bronchiolitis obliterans
bucc(o)-	Of or pertaining to the cheek	Buccolabial
burs(o)-	bursa (fluid sac between the bones)	Bursitis

Anatomy and Physiology for Nursing and Healthcare Students at a Glance, Second Edition. Ian Peate.
© 2022 John Wiley & Sons Ltd. Published 2022 by John Wiley & Sons Ltd.
Companion website: www.wiley.com/go/peate/anatomyandphysiology

Prefix or suffix	Meaning	Example(s)
carcin(o)-	cancer	Carcinoma
cardi(o)-	Of or pertaining to the heart	Cardiology
carp(o)-	Of or pertaining to the wrist	Carpopedal
-cele	pouching, hernia	Hydrocele, Varicocele
-centesis	surgical puncture for aspiration	Amniocentesis
cephal(o)-	Of or pertaining to the head (as a whole)	Cephalalgy
cerebell(o)-	Of or pertaining to the cerebellum	Cerebellum
cerebr(o)-	Of or pertaining to the brain	Cerebrology
chem(o)-	chemistry, drug	Chemotherapy
chol(e)-	Of or pertaining to bile	Cholecystitis
cholecyst(o)-	Of or pertaining to the gallbladder	Cholecystectomy
chondr(i)o-	cartilage, gristle, granule, granular	Chondrocalcinosis
chrom(ato)-	colour	Haemochromatosis
-cidal, -cide	killing, destroying	Bacteriocidal
cili-	Of or pertaining to the cilia, the eyelashes; eyelids	Ciliary
circum-	Denoting something as 'around' another	Circumcision
col-, colo-, colono-	colon	Colonoscopy
colp(o)-	Of or pertaining to the vagina	Colposcopy
contra	against	Contraindicate
coron(o)-	crown	Coronary
cost(o)-	Of or pertaining to the ribs	Costochondral
crani(o)-	Belonging or relating to the cranium	Craniology
-crine, crin(o)	to secrete	Endocrine
cry(o)-	cold	Cryoablation
cutane-	skin	Subcutaneous
cyan(o)-	Denotes a blue color	Cyanopsia
cyst(o)-, cyst(i)-	Of or pertaining to the urinary bladder	Cystotomy
cyt(o)-	cell	Cytokine
-cyte	cell	Leukocyte

-dactyl(o)-	Of or pertaining to a finger, toe	Dactylology, polydactyly
dent-	Of or pertaining to teeth	Dentist
dermat(o)-, derm(o)-	Of or pertaining to the skin	Dermatology
-desis	binding	Arthrodesis
dextr(o)-	right, on the right side	Dextrocardia
di-	two	Diplopia
dia-	through, during, across	Dialysis
dif-	apart, separation	Different
digit-	Of or pertaining to the finger [rare as a root]	Digit
-dipsia	Suffix meaning '(condition of) thirst'	Polydipsia, hydroadipsia, oligodipsia
dors(o)-, dors(i)-	Of or pertaining to the back	Dorsal, dorsocephalad
duodeno-	duodenum, upper part of the small intestine (twelve inches long on average), connects to the stomach	Duodenal atresia
dynam(o)-	force, energy, power	Hand strength dynamometer
-dynia	pain	Vulvodynia
dys-	bad, difficult, defective, abnormal	Dysphagia, dysphasia

ec-	out, away	Ectopia, ectopic pregnancy
ect(o)-	outer, outside	Ectoblast, ectoderm
-ectasia, -ectasis	expansion, dilation	Bronchiectasis, telangiectasia
-ectomy	Denotes a surgical operation or removal of a body part. Resection, excision	Mastectomy
-emesis	vomiting condition	Haematemesis
-aemia	blood condition	Anaemia
encephal(o)-	Of or pertaining to the brain. Also see Cerebro	Encephalogram
endo-	Denotes something as 'inside' or 'within'	Endocrinology, endospore
eosin (o)-	Red	Eosinophil granulocyte
enter(o)-	Of or pertaining to the intestine	Gastroenterology
epi-	on, upon	Epicardium, epidermis, epidural, episclera, epistaxis
erythr(o)-	Denotes a red colour	Erythrocyte
ex-	out of, away from	Excision, exophthalmos
exo-	Denotes something as 'outside' another	Exoskeleton
extra-	outside	Extradural haematoma

Prefix or suffix	Meaning	Example(s)
faci(o)-	Of or pertaining to the face	Facioplegic
fibr(o)	fibre	Fibroblast
fore-	before or ahead	Foreword
fossa	A hollow or depressed area; trench or channel	Fossa ovalis
front-	Of or pertaining to the forehead	Frontonasal
galact(o)-	milk	Galactorrhoea
gastr(o)-	Of or pertaining to the stomach	Gastric bypass
-genic	Formative, pertaining to producing	Cardiogenic shock
gingiv-	Of or pertaining to the gums	Gingivitis
glauc(o)-	Denoting a grey or bluish-grey colour	Glaucoma
gloss(o)-, glott(o)-	Of or pertaining to the tongue	Glossology
gluco-	sweet	Glucocorticoid
glyc(o)-	sugar	Glycolysis
-gnosis	knowledge	Diagnosis, prognosis
gon(o)-	seed, semen; also, reproductive	Gonorrhoea
-gram, -gramme	record or picture	Angiogram
-graph	instrument used to record data or picture	Electrocardiograph
-graphy	process of recording	Angiography
gyn(aec)o-	woman	Gynaecomastia
halluc-	to wander in mind	Hallucinosis
haemat-, haemato- (haem-,)	Of or pertaining to blood	Haematology
haemangi or haemangio-	blood vessels	Haemangioma
hemi-	one-half	Cerebral hemisphere
hepat- (hepatic-)	Of or pertaining to the liver	Hepatology
heter(o)-	Denotes something as 'the other' (of two), as an addition, or different	Heterogeneous
hist(o)-, histio-	tissue	Histology
home(o)-	similar	Homeopathy
hom(o)-	Denotes something as 'the same' as another or common	Homosexuality
hydr(o)-	water	Hydrophobe
hyper-	Denotes something as 'extreme' or 'beyond normal'	Hypertension
hyp(o)-	Denotes something as 'below normal'	Hypovolaemia
hyster(o)-	Of or pertaining to the womb, the uterus	Hysterectomy, hysteria
iatr(o)-	Of or pertaining to medicine, or a physician	Iatrogenic
-iatry	Denotes a field in medicine of a certain body component	Podiatry, Psychiatry
-ics	organised knowledge, treatment	Obstetrics
ileo-	ileum	Ileocecal valve
infra-	below	Infrahyoid muscles
inter-	between, among	Interarticular ligament
intra-	within	Intramural
ipsi-	same	Ipsilateral hemiparesis
ischio-	Of or pertaining to the ischium, the hip-joint	Ischioanal fossa
-ism	condition, disease	Dwarfism
-ismus	spasm, contraction	Hemiballismus
iso-	Denoting something as being 'equal'	Isotonic
-ist	one who specialises in	Pathologist
-itis	inflammation	Tonsillitis
-ium	structure, tissue	Pericardium
Juxta (iuxta)	Near to, alongside or next to	Juxtaglomerular apparatus
karyo-	nucleus	Eukaryote
kerat(o)-	cornea (eye or skin)	Keratoscope
kin(e)-, kin(o), kinesi(o)-	movement	Kinesthaesia
kyph(o)-	humped	Kyphoscoliosis
labi(o)-	Of or pertaining to the lip	Labiodental
lacrim(o)-	tear	Lacrimal canaliculi
lact(i)-, lact(o)	milk	Lactation
lapar(o)-	Of or pertaining to the abdomen-wall, flank	Laparotomy

Prefix or suffix	Meaning	Example(s)
laryng(o)-	Of or pertaining to the larynx, the lower throat cavity where the voice box is	Larynx
latero-	lateral	Lateral pectoral nerve
-lepsis, -lepsy	attack, seizure	Epilepsy, narcolepsy
lept(o)-	light, slender	Leptomeningeal
leuc(o)-, leuk(o)-	Denoting a white colour	Leukocyte
lingu(a)-, lingu(o)-	Of or pertaining to the tongue	Linguistics
lip(o)-	fat	Liposuction
lith(o)-	stone, calculus	Lithotripsy
log(o)-	speech	
-logist	Denotes someone who studies a certain field	Oncologist, pathologist
-logy	Denotes the academic study or practice of a certain field	Haematology, urology
lymph(o)-	lymph	Lymphoedema
lys(o)-, -lytic	dissolution	Lysosome
-lysis	Destruction, separation	Paralysis
macr(o)-	large, long	Macrophage
-malacia	softening	Osteomalacia
mamm(o)-	Of or pertaining to the breast	Mammogram
mammill(o)-	Of or pertaining to the nipple	Mammillaplasty, mammillitis
manu-	Of or pertaining to the hand	Manufacture
mast(o)-	Of or pertaining to the breast	Mastectomy
meg(a)-, megal(o)-, -megaly	enlargement, million	Splenomegaly, megameter
melan(o)-	black colour	Melanin
mening(o)-	membrane	Meningitis
meta-	after, behind	Metacarpus
-meter	Instrument used to measure or count	Sphygmomanometer
-metry	process of measuring	Optometry
metr(o)-	Pertaining to conditions or instruments of the uterus	Metrorrhagia
micro-	Denoting something as small, or relating to smallness, millionth	Microscope
milli-	thousandth	Millilitre
mon(o)-	single	Infectious mononucleosis
morph(o)-	form, shape	Morphology
muscul(o)-	muscle	Musculoskeletal system
my(o)-	Of or relating to muscle	Myoblast
myc(o)-	fungus	Onychomycosis
myel(o)-	Of or relating to bone marrow or spinal cord	Myeloblast
myri-	ten thousand	Myriad
myring(o)-	eardrum	Myringotomy
narc(o)-	numb, sleep	Narcolepsy
nas(o)-	Of or pertaining to the nose	Nasal
necr(o)-	death	Necrosis, necrotising fasciitis
neo-	new	Neoplasm
nephr(o)-	Of or pertaining to the kidney	Nephrology
neur(i)-, neur(o)-	Of or pertaining to nerves and the nervous system	Neurofibromatosis
normo-	normal	Normocapnia
ocul(o)-	Of or pertaining to the eye	Oculist
odont(o)-	Of or pertaining to teeth	Orthodontist
odyn(o)-	pain	Stomatodynia
-oesophageal, oesophago-	gullet	Oesophagogastrectomy
-oesophageal, -oesophago-	gullet	Oesophagus
-oid	resemblance to	Sarcoidosis
ole	small or little	Micromole
olig(o)-	Denoting something as 'having little, having few'	Oliguria
-oma (singular), -omata (plural)	tumour, mass, collection	Sarcoma, teratoma
onco-	tumour, bulk, volume	Oncology
onych(o)-	Of or pertaining to the nail (of a finger or toe)	Onychophagy
oo-	Of or pertaining to the an egg, a woman's egg, the ovum	Oogenesis
oophor(o)-	Of or pertaining to the woman's ovary	Oophorectomy

Prefix or suffix	Meaning	Example(s)
ophthalm(o)-	Of or pertaining to the eye	Ophthalmology
optic(o)-	Of or relating to chemical properties of the eye	Opticochemical,
orchi(o)-, orchid(o)-, orch(o)-	testes	Orchiectomy, orchidectomy
-osis	A condition, disease or increase	Harlequin type ichthyosis, psychosis, osteoperosis
osseo-	bony	Osseous
ossi-	bone	Peripheral ossifying fibroma
ost(e)-, oste(o)-	bone	Osteoporosis
ot(o)-	Of or pertaining to the ear	Otology
ovo-, ovi-, ov-	Of or pertaining to the eggs, the ovum	Ovogenesis
oxo-	addition of oxygen	

Prefix or suffix	Meaning	Example(s)
pachy-	thick	Pachyderma
palpebr-	Of or pertaining to the eyelid [uncommon as a root]	Palpebra
pan-, pant(o)-	Denoting something as 'complete' or containing 'everything'	Panophobia, panopticon
papill-	Of or pertaining to the nipple (of the chest/breast)	Papillitis
papul(o)-	Indicates papulosity, a small elevation or swelling in the skin, a pimple, swelling	Papulation
para-	alongside of, abnormal	Paracyesis
-paresis	slight paralysis	Hemiparesis
parvo-	small	Parvovirus
path(o)-	disease	Pathology
-pathy	Denotes (with a negative sense) a disease, or disorder	Sociopathy, neuropathy
pector-	breast	Pectoralgia, pectoriloquy, pectorophony
ped-, -ped-, -pes	Of or pertaining to the foot; -footed	Pedoscope
ped-, pedo-	Of or pertaining to the child	Paediatrics paedophilia
pelv(i)-, pelv(o)-	hip bone	Pelvis
-penia	deficiency	Osteopenia
-pepsia	Denotes something relating to digestion, or the digestive tract	Dyspepsia
peri-	Denoting something with a position 'surrounding' or 'around' another	Periodontal
-pexy	fixation	Nephropexy
phaco-	lens-shaped	Phacolysis, phacometer, phacoscotoma
-phage, -phagia	Forms terms denoting conditions relating to eating or ingestion	Sarcophagia
-phago-	eating, devouring	Phagocyte
phagist-:	Forms nouns that denote a person who 'feeds on' the first element or part of the word	Lotophagi
-phagy	Forms nouns that denotes 'feeding on' the first element or part of the word	Haematophagy
pharmaco-	drug, medication	Pharmacology
pharyng(o)-	Of or pertaining to the pharynx, the upper throat cavity	Pharyngitis, Pharyngoscopy
phleb(o)-	Of or pertaining to the (blood) veins, a vein	Phlebography, Phlebotomy
-phobia	exaggerated fear, sensitivity	Arachnophobia
phon(o)-	sound	Phonograph, symphony
phos-	Of or pertaining to light or its chemical properties, now historic and used rarely. See the common root phot(o)- below	Phosphene
phot(o)-	Of or pertaining to light	Photopathy
phren(i)-, phren(o)-, phrenico	the mind	Phrenic nerve, schizophrenia
-plasia	formation, development	Achondroplasia
-plasty	surgical repair, reconstruction	Rhinoplasty
-plegia	paralysis	Paraplegia
pleio-	more, excessive, multiple	Pleiomorphism
pleur(o)-, pleur(a)	Of or pertaining to the ribs	Pleurogenous
-plexy	stroke or seizure	Cataplexy
pneum(o)-	Of or pertaining to the lungs	Pneumonocyte, Pneumonia Pneumatosis, Pneumatic
-poiesis	production	Haematopoiesis
poly-	Denotes a 'plurality' of something	Polymyositis
post-	Denotes something as 'after' or 'behind' another	Postoperation, Postmortem
pre-	Denotes something as 'before' another (in [physical] position or time)	Premature birth
presby(o)-	old age	Presbyopia
prim-	Denotes something as 'first' or 'most-important'	Primary
proct(o)-	anus, rectum	Proctology
prot(o)-	Denotes something as 'first' or 'most important'	Protoneuron
pseud(o)-	Denotes something false or fake	Pseudoephedrine

Prefix or suffix	Meaning	Example(s)
psych(e)-, psych(o)	Of or pertaining to the mind	Psychology, psychiatry
psor-	itching	Psoriasis
-ptosis	falling, drooping, downward placement, prolapse	Apoptosis, nephroptosis
-ptysis	(a spitting), spitting, haemoptysis, the spitting of blood derived from the lungs or bronchial tubes	Haemoptysis
pulmon-, pulmo-	Of or relating to the lungs.	Pulmonary
pyel(o)-	pelvis	Pyelonephritis
py(o)-	pus	Pyometra
pyr(o)-	fever	Antipyretic

quadr(i)-	four	Quadriceps

radio-	radiation	Radiowave
ren(o)-	Of or pertaining to the kidney	Renal
retro-	backward, behind	Retroversion, retroverted
rhin(o)-	Of or pertaining to the nose	Rhinoplasty
rhod(o)-	Denoting a rose-red colour	Rhodophyte
-rrhage	burst forth	Haemorrhage
-rrhagia	rapid flow of blood	Menorrhagia
-rrhaphy	surgical suturing	Herniorraphy
-rrhexis	rupture	Karyorrhexis
-rrhoea	flowing, discharge	Diarrhoea
-rupt	Break or burst	Erupt, interrupt

salping(o)-	Of or pertaining to tubes, e.g. fallopian tubes	Salpingectomy, salpingopharyngeus muscle
sangui-, sanguine-	Of or pertaining to blood	Sanguine
sarco-	muscular, flesh-like	Sarcoma
scler(o)-	hard	Scleroderma
-sclerosis	hardening	Atherosclerosis, multiple sclerosis
scoli(o)-	twisted	Scoliosis
-scope	instrument for viewing	Otoscope
-scopy	use of instrument for viewing	Endoscopy
semi-	one-half, partly	Semiconscious
sial(o)-	saliva, salivary gland	Sialagogue
sigmoid(o)-	sigmoid, S-shaped curvature	Sigmoid colon
sinus-	Of or pertaining to the sinus	Sinusitis
somat(o)-, somatico-	body, bodily	Somatic
-spadias	slit, fissure	Hypospadias, epispadias
spasmo-	spasm	Spasmodic dysphonia
sperma-, spermo-, spermato-	semen, spermatozoa	Spermatogenesis
splen(o)-	spleen	Splenectomy
spondyl(o)-	Of or pertaining to the spine, the vertebra	Spondylitis
squamos(o)-	Denoting something as 'full of scales' or 'scaly'	Squamous cell
-stalsis	contraction	Peristalsis
-stasis	stopping, standing	Cytostasis, homeostasis
-staxis	dripping, trickling	Epistaxis
-stenosis	abnormal narrowing in a blood vessel or other tubular organ or structure	Restenosis, stenosis
stomat(o)-	Of or pertaining to the mouth	Stomatogastric, stomatognathic system
-stomy	creation of an opening	Colostomy
sub-	beneath	Subcutaneous tissue
super-	in excess, above, superior	Superior vena cava
supra-	above, excessive	Supraorbital vein

tachy-	Denoting something as fast, irregularly fast	Tachycardia
-tension, -tensive	pressure	Hypertension
tetan-	rigid, tense	Tetanus
thec-	case, sheath	Intrathecal
therap-	treatment	Hydrotherapy, therapeutic
therm(o)-	heat	Thermometer
thorac(i)-, thorac(o)-, thoracico-	Of or pertaining to the upper chest, chest; the area above the breast and under the neck	Thoracic
thromb(o)-	Of or relating to a blood clot, clotting of blood	Thrombus, thrombocytopenia

Prefix or suffix	Meaning	Example(s)
thyr(o)-	thyroid	Thyroidism
thym-	emotions	Dysthymia
-tome	cutting instrument	Dermatome
-tomy	act of cutting; incising, incision	Gastrotomy
tono-	tone, tension, pressure	Tonometry
-tony	tension	Tonicity
top(o)-	place, topical	Topical anaesthetic
tort(i)-	twisted	Torticollis
tox(i)-, tox(o)-, toxic(o)-	toxin, poison	Toxoplasmosis
trache(a)-	trachea	Tracheotomy
trachel(o)-	Of or pertaining to the neck	Tracheloplasty
trans-	Denoting something as moving or situated 'across' or 'through'	Transfusion
tri-	three	Triangle
trich(i)-, trichia, trich(o)-	Of or pertaining to hair, hair-like structure	Trichocyst
-tripsy	crushing	Lithotripsy
-trophy	nourishment, development	Pseudohypertrophy
tympan(o)-	eardrum	Tympanocentesis
-ula, -ule	small	Nodule
ultra-	beyond, excessive	Ultrasound
un(i)-	one	Unilateral hearing loss
ur(o)-	Of or pertaining to urine, the urinary system; (specifically) pertaining to the physiological chemistry of urine	Urology
uter(o)-	Of or pertaining to the uterus or womb	Uterus
vagin-	Of or pertaining to the vagina	Vagina
varic(o)-	swollen or twisted vein	Varicose
vas(o)-	duct, blood vessel	Vasoconstriction
vasculo-	blood vessel	Vasculogenic
ven-	Of or pertaining to the (blood) veins, a vein (*used in terms pertaining to the vascular system*)	Vein, Venospasm
ventr(o)-	Of or pertaining to the abdomen; the stomachcavities	Ventrodorsal
ventricul(o)-	Of or pertaining to the ventricles; any hollow region inside an organ	Cardiac ventriculography
-version	turning	Anteversion, retroversion
vesic(o)-	Of or pertaining to the bladder	Vesical arteries
viscer(o)-	Of or pertaining to the internal organs, the viscera	Viscera
xanth(o)-	Denoting a yellow colour, an abnormally yellow colour	Xanthopathy
xen(o)-	foreign, different	Xenograft
xer(o)-	dry, desert-like	Xerostomia
zo(o)-	animal, animal life	Zoology
zym(o)-	fermentation	Enzyme, lysozyme

Appendix 3: Glossary

Absorption: The transport of molecules across epithelial membranes into the body fluids

Acinus: Saliva secreting cluster of cells

Acromegaly: Excessive growth due to the production of excessive growth hormone by the pituitary gland

Active immunity: Immunity involving sensitisation, in which antibody production is stimulated by prior exposure to an antigen.

Adenine: One of the four nitrogen-carbon bases of DNA

Adipose cells: Groups of fat cells forming yellow lobules in subcutaneous tissue

ADH: Hormone produced by the hypothalamus and stored in the posterior pituitary gland

Afferent: Conveying or transmitting to

Allergy: Hypersensitivity caused by exposure to allergens, resulting in the release of histamine and other molecules with similar histamine effects

Anaemia: A condition whereby there is a lack of red blood cells

Anterior: In front of

Antibodies: Substances made by the body's immune system in response, for example, to bacteria, viruses, fungus or cancer cells.

Antigens: A substance that when introduced into the body stimulates antibody production.

Anuria: Without the formation of urine

Apnoea: Cessation of breathing

Aquaporins: Transmembrane proteins that aid water reabsorption

Arthralgia: Pain in a joint

Arthroplasty: Surgical replacement of a joint

Aural: Pertaining to the ear

Atrioventricular node: A section of nodal tissue that lies on the right side of the partition that divides the atria, near the bottom of the right atrium

Atrioventricular valves: Collective name of the two valves that lie between the atria and the ventricles

Axilla: The armpit

Axon: Process of a neuron that carries impulses away from the body

Azoospermia: A condition in which there is a lack of spermatozoa in the semen

Baroreceptors: Sensors located in the blood vessels

Bronchodilation: Expansion of the bronchial air passages

Calcitonin: A hormone secreted by the thyroid gland which controls the levels of calcium and phosphorous in the blood

Cancellous bone: Synonymous with trabecular bone or spongy bone, one of two types of osseous tissue forming bones. The other is cortical bone

Cancer: A tumour characterised by abnormally rapid cell division and the loss of specialised tissue characteristics, usually refers to malignant tumours

Capillaries: Tiny blood vessels

Cardiac cycle: The sequence of events that occurs when the heart beats

Cardiac muscle: Muscle of the heart, consisting of striated muscle cells that are interconnected into a mass called the myocardium

Catabolism: The metabolic breakdown of complex molecules into simpler ones, often resulting in a release of energy

Cations: Positively charged ions

Cell membrane: Outer layer of the cell

Cerebrum: The largest anatomical structure of the brain

Cerebellum: Portion of the brain responsible for coordinated and smooth muscle movements

Ceruminous glands: A specialised integumentary gland secreting cerumen, (or earwax) into the external auditory canal

Chemokines: A family of small cytokines, or signalling proteins secreted by cells

Chemoreceptor: A neuroreceptor that is stimulated by the presence of chemical molecules

Cholinergic: Denoting nerve endings that liberate acetylcholine as a neurotransmitter, such as those of the parasympathetic nervous system

Chromosome: Mixture of DNA and protein

Chyme: Creamy, semi fluid mass of partially digested food mixed with gastric secretions

Cochlea: The organ of hearing in the inner ear where nerve impulses are generated in response to sound waves.

Conchal surface: A long, narrow and curled bone shelf (shaped like an elongated sea-shell) that protrudes into the breathing passage of the nose

Conjugated bile: Formed by the union of two compounds

Corpus: The main body or mass of a structure

Cortex: The outer aspect of an organ

Corticosteroids: Hormones produced by the adrenal gland, consisting of hydrocortisone (or cortisol)

Cryptorchidism: Developmental defect in which one or both testes fail to descend into the scrotum

Cyanosis: A dark blue condition of the skin and mucous membranes caused by oxygen deficiency

Cytoplasm: Fluid found inside the cell

Cytosine: One of the four nitrogen-carbon bases of DNA

Decussation: Crossing over of neurons

Diaphysis: The shaft of a long bone

Diastolic phase: The relaxation phase when the chambers of the heart fill with blood

Diffusion: The passive movement of molecules or ions from a region of high concentration to low concentration until a state of equilibrium is achieved

Digestion: The chemical and mechanical breakdown of food for absorption

Diplopia: Double vision

Diuresis: Excess urine production

Dura mater: The outermost of the three layers of the meninges that surround the brain and spinal cord

Efferent: Conveying away from the centre of an organ or structure

Effector: A muscle, gland, or organ capable of responding to a stimulus, especially a nerve impulse

Electrolytes: An electrolyte is a compound that ionises when dissolved in suitable ionising solvents such as water

Endo: Internal or within

Endocardium: Inner layer of the heart that lines the chambers and the valves

Anatomy and Physiology for Nursing and Healthcare Students at a Glance, Second Edition. Ian Peate.
© 2022 John Wiley & Sons Ltd. Published 2022 by John Wiley & Sons Ltd.
Companion website: www.wiley.com/go/peate/anatomyandphysiology

Endocrine: Glands which secrete hormones directly into the bloodstream

Endocytosis: An energy-using process by which cells absorb molecules (such as proteins) by engulfing them

Endometrium: Lining of the uterus

Enzymes: Biological catalysts – catalysts are substances that increase the rate of chemical reactions without being used up

Epinephrine: Adrenaline

Epiphysis: The end segment of a long bone, separated from the diaphysis early in life by an epiphyseal plate, later this becomes part of the larger bone

Ethmoid bones: A bone in the skull that separates the nasal cavity from the brain

Extracellular matrix: Any substance produced by cells and excreted to the extracellular space within the tissues, serving as a scaffolding to hold tissues together and helping to determine their characteristics

Exocrine: Glands which secrete hormones into ducts

Exocytosis: The process in which the cell releases materials to the outside by discharging them as membrane-bounded vesicles passing through the cell membrane

Filtration: Passive transport system

Follicle: A small secretory cavity, sac, or gland

Ganglia: A group of neuronal cell bodies lying outside the CNS

Gene: A unit of heredity in a living organism

Gingiva: The fleshy covering over the mandible and maxilla through which the teeth protrude within the mouth

Glucagon: A peptide hormone secreted by the pancreas, raises blood glucose levels

Glycogenesis: The formation of glycogen, the primary carbohydrate stored in the liver and muscle cells

Glomerulus: A network of capillaries found in the Bowman's capsule

Gluconeogenesis: The creation of glucose from non-carbohydrate molecules

Glycolysis: The anaerobic breakdown of glucose to form pyruvic acid

Gonad: A reproductive organ, testes or ovary, producing gametes and sex hormones

Guanine: One of the four nitrogen-carbon bases of DNA

Haemopoiesis: A biological process in which new blood cells are formed, which usually takes place in the bone marrow

Hilum: A small indented part of the kidney

Hirsuitism: Excessive growth of body and facial hair, including the chest, stomach and back

Histamine: A compound secreted by tissue mast cells and other connective tissue cells that stimulates vasodilation and increases capillary permeability

Homeostasis: The tendency of an organism or a cell to regulate its internal conditions, usually by a system of feedback controls, so as to stabilise health and functioning, regardless of the outside changing conditions

Hyaline cartilage: A translucent bluish-white type of cartilage present in the joints as well as the respiratory tract and the immature skeleton

Hydrophilic: Water-loving

Hydrophobic: Water-hating

Hypercapnia: A condition where there is too much carbon dioxide in the blood.

Hypoxia: Term used when a cell or tissue is deprived of oxygen

IgA: Antibodies are found in areas of the body such the nose, breathing passages, digestive tract, ears, eyes and vagina

IgD: Antibodies found in small amounts in the tissues that line the chest

IgE: Antibodies found in the lungs, skin, and mucous membranes

IgG: Antibodies found in all body fluids

IgM: The largest antibody

Immunocompetent: Having a normal immune response

Incus: The middle of three auditory ossicles within the middle-ear chamber (anvil)

Inferior: Below

Inferolateral: Located below and towards the side

Insulin: A peptide hormone, produced by beta cells of the pancreas, it regulates carbohydrate and fat metabolism in the body

Ischaemia: Inadequate blood supply to an organ or part of the body, especially the heart muscles

Isthmus: A narrow organ, passage, or piece of tissue connecting two larger parts.

Juxtaglomerular cells: A microscopic structure in the kidney, which regulates the function of each nephron

Keratin: An insoluble protein present in the epidermis and in epidermal derivatives, such as hair and nails

Labyrinth: An intricate structure consisting of interconnecting passages, for example, the bony and membranous labyrinths of the inner ear

Lactation: The production and secretion of milk by the mammary glands

Lacuna: A small, hollow chamber housing an osteocyte in mature bone tissue or a chondrocyte in cartilage tissue

Lamella: Concentric ring of matrix surrounding the central canal in an osteon of mature bone tissue

Lateral: To the side

Lesion: A wounded or damaged area

Libido: Sexual desire

Ligament: A short band of tough, flexible fibrous connective tissue connecting two bones or cartilages, or holding together a joint

Limbic system: Limbic system structures are involved in many of our emotions and motivations, particularly those that are related to survival

Lipogenesis: The process by which simple sugars such as glucose are converted to fatty acids

Locomotion: Movement

Lymphocytes: White blood cells

Lysosyme: Cellular organelles that contain acid hydrolase enzymes that break down waste materials and cellular debris

Macrophages: White blood cells within tissues, produced by the division of monocytes

Mast cell: A type of connective tissue cell producing and secreting histamine and heparin and promoting local inflammation.

Malleus: The first of three auditory ossicles that attaches to the tympanum (the hammer)

Medial: Toward the centre

Medulla: The inner region of an organ or tissue, particularly when distinct from the outer region or cortex (for example, a kidney, an adrenal gland)

Meiosis: A process in which diploid cells become haploid cells, thus ensuring correct number of chromosomes are passed on to offspring

Melatonin: Hormone secreted by the pineal gland, produces lightening of the skin

Menarche: The first menstrual discharge

Meninges: Three layers of tissue that cover and protect the CNS

Metabolism: Sum total of the chemical reactions occurring in the body

Mitosis: A process by which chromosomes are accurately reproduced in cells during cell division

Myocardium: Muscle layer of the heart

Nasal septum: Bony and cartilaginous partition separating the nasal cavity into two portions.

Node of Ranvier: Periodic gap in the insulating sheath (myelin) on the axon of certain neurons that serves to facilitate the rapid conduction of nerve impulses

Norepinephrine: Noradrenaline

Nephron: Functional units of the kidney

Neuromuscular junction: The junction between a nerve fibre and the muscle it supplies

Neurotransmitters: chemical messengers

Olfactory: Pertaining to the sense of smell

Oocyte: A cell in an ovary which may undergo meiotic division to form an ovum

Optic: Pertaining to the eye

Os: Opening

Osteoblast: A bone-forming cell

Osteoclast: A cell that causes erosion and resorption of bone tissue

Osteocyte: A mature bone cell

Osteons: Or Haversian system; the fundamental functional unit of compact bone

Ossification: The process of bone formation

Ovarian ligament: A cordlike connective tissue attaching the ovary to the uterus

Ovulation: The rupture of an ovarian (graafian) follicle with the release of an ovum

Oxytocin: Hormone that stimulates contractions of the uterus during labour

Palpebra: An eyelid

Papillae: Nipple like structure on the tongue that gives it its rough texture

Pericardium: Double layered sac that surrounds the heart

Perilymph: A fluid of the inner ear providing a liquid-conducting medium for the vibrations involved in hearing and equilibrium

Periosteum: A fibrous connective tissue covering the outer surface of bone

Peripheral resistance: The force against blood flow in a blood vessel

Peristalsis: Wave-like contractions that move food through the digestive tract

Phagocytosis: The process of engulfing and ingestion of particles by the cell or a phagocyte such as a macrophage

Pia mater: Innermost layer of the meninges

Pinna: The outer, fleshy portion of the external ear; also known as the auricle

Pinocytosis: A process by which the cell takes in the fluids along with dissolved small molecules.

Polysaccharides: Long carbohydrate molecules of monosaccharide units joined together by glycosidic bonds

Posterior: Behind

Pneumotaxic area: This area is in the pons and is important for regulating the amount of air one takes in with each breath

Pulmonary circulation: A short circulation from the right ventricle to the lungs and back to the heart

Pulmonary ventilation: The process by which gases are exchanged between atmospheric air and the lungs

Raphe: A ridge or a seam-like structure between two similar parts of a body organ; for example, the scrotum

Receptor: A specialised cell or group of nerve endings that responds to sensory stimuli

Renal cortex: The outer most part of the kidney

Renal medulla: The middle part of the kidney

Renal pelvis: The funnel-shaped section of the kidney

Renal pyramids: Cone-shaped structures of the medulla

Ribosomes: Small bead-like structures in a cell, along with RNA, are involved in making proteins from amino acids

Rugae: The folds or ridges of the mucosa of an organ

Sarcolemma: The membrane covering a striated muscle

Sarcoplasm: The cytoplasm of striated muscle cells.

SA node: The pacemaker of the heart

Sebum: An oily, waterproofing secretion of the sebaceous glands

Semicircular canals: Tubule channels within the inner ear containing receptors for equilibrium.

Sensory nerves: Neurones that carry sensory information from the cranial and spinal nerves into the brain and the spinal cord

Serum: Blood plasma with the clotting elements removed

Septum: Dividing wall of the heart

Somatic nervous system: Voluntary motor division of the peripheral nervous system

Spectrin: A cytoskeletal protein that lines the intracellular side of the plasma membrane

Spermatogenesis: The production or development of mature spermatozoa

Sphincter: A ring-like muscle fibre that can constrict

Stapes: The innermost of the auditory ossicles that fits against the oval window of the inner ear (the stirrup)

Superior: Above

Systemic circulation: Flow of blood from the left ventricle to the whole body

Systolic phase: The phase when the chambers of the heart are actively pumping the blood

Tendon: A band of dense regular connective tissue attaching muscle to bone

Thyroxine (T_4): A hormone secreted by the thyroid gland which regulates metabolism

Triiodothyronine (T_3): A hormone secreted by the thyroid gland which regulates metabolism

Thrombocytes: Cells that play a role in blood clotting

Thymine: One of the four nitrogen-carbon bases of DNA

Thymosins: Small proteins present in many animal tissues. So called because they originate from the thymus gland

Trabeculae: A supporting framework of fibres crossing the substance of a structure, as in the lamellae of spongy bone

Tympanic membrane: The membranous eardrum positioned between the external and middle ear

Unmyelinated: Not covered by myelin sheath

Ureter: Membranous tube that drains urine from the kidneys to the bladder

Urethra: Muscular tube that drains urine from the bladder

Vasodilate: Dilation of blood vessels

Vasoconstrict: Constriction of the blood vessels

Visceral: Pertaining to internal organs of the body

Vomer: One of the unpaired facial bones of the skull

White matter: Myelinated nerve fibres

Zygote: A fertilised egg cell formed by the union of a sperm cell and an ovum

Further reading

Gilroy, A.M. (2013) *Anatomy: An Essential Text Book*. Thieme: New York.

Hankin, M., Morse, D. and Bennett-Clarke, C. (2013) *Clinical Anatomy: A Case Study Approach*. McGraw-Hill: New York.

Jenkins, G.W. and Tortora, G.J. (2013) *Anatomy and Physiology: From Science to Life*, 3rd edn. Wiley: New Jersey.

Martini, F.H. (2016) *Essentials of Anatomy and Physiology*, 7th edn. Pearson: New York.

Patton, K.Y. and Thibodeau, G.A. (2013) *The Human Body in Health and Disease*, 6th edn. Elsevier: St Louis.

Peate, I. (2021) *Fundamentals of Applied Pathophysiology for Nursing and Healthcare Students*. 4th edn. Wiley: Oxford.

Peate, I. and Evans, S. (eds) (2020) *Fundamentals of Anatomy and Physiology for Student Nurses*. 3rd edn. Wiley: Oxford.

Tortora, G.J. (2013) *Principles of Anatomy and Physiology*, 14th edn. Wiley: New Jersey.

Index

Anatomy and Physiology for Nursing and Healthcare Students at a Glance, Second Edition. Ian Peate.
© 2022 John Wiley & Sons Ltd. Published 2022 by John Wiley & Sons Ltd.
Companion website: www.wiley.com/go/peate/anatomyandphysiology